PENGUIN BOOKS

The Criminal Mind

Dr Duncan Harding is a consultant adolescent forensic psychiatrist, working with adults and children who commit serious crime. He is a specialist member of the Parole Board for England and Wales, and the college lead for expert witnesses at the Royal College of Psychiatrists. Specializing in forensic mental health, he has provided expert testimony in many court cases involving homicide, serious violence and terrorism, and has conducted research into conduct disorder and criminal psychopathy. He lives in London.

The Criminal Mind

DR DUNCAN HARDING

PENGUIN BOOKS

PENGUIN BOOKS

UK | USA | Canada | Ireland | Australia
India | New Zealand | South Africa

Penguin Books is part of the Penguin Random House group of companies
whose addresses can be found at global.penguinrandomhouse.com

Penguin Random House UK,
One Embassy Gardens, 8 Viaduct Gardens, London SW11 7BW

penguin.co.uk

First published by Penguin Michael Joseph 2024
Published by Penguin Books 2025
003

Typeset by Jouve (UK), Milton Keynes
Printed and bound in Great Britain by Clays Ltd, Elcograf S.p.A.

The authorized representative in the EEA is Penguin Random House Ireland,
Morrison Chambers, 32 Nassau Street, Dublin D02 YH68

A CIP catalogue record for this book is available from the British Library

ISBN: 978–1–405–94561–5

Penguin Random House is committed to a sustainable future
for our business, our readers and our planet. This book is made from
Forest Stewardship Council® certified paper.

MIX
Paper | Supporting responsible forestry
FSC® C018179

For my dear mum, Dorothy

Author's Note

My work has given me unparalleled access to patients, their relatives, and the human condition in general. Such access is privileged and sacrosanct. This book is a collection of my thoughts and professional opinions. Respect for patient confidentiality is extremely important, for me and any doctor, and I have changed key facts and details to protect confidentiality. The facts are a scaffolding used to frame the cases; the insights and opinions are my own. Indeed, these cases are an amalgam of different encounters and experiences – I have at times changed gender, age, place and circumstances to protect the privacy of others.

In context, at the time of writing this book, the UK is gripped in a knife crime and murder epidemic. Children kill other children almost every weekend. What has happened to cause this? Why are our disenfranchised youth destroying the life and beauty that surround them in this fragile and precious world? I feel it is my duty to talk about this, to open the lid on heartbreaking cases and situations, to try to understand these extreme patterns of behaviour.

So, after a lot of thought and discussion with senior colleagues, I decided to write this book. I hope it does no harm. I hope it is useful.

I

'I'm phoning to report a death. In fact, it's a murder.'

The voice was young and matter-of-fact.

'I see,' said the call handler flatly. He gave no indication of surprise. Perhaps he received calls like this every day. 'And can you tell me who's been murdered?'

'My aunt. I killed her.'

'Are you sure she's dead?'

'Yeah, she's really, really dead.'

It was hard to guess who sounded less bothered: Liam, the seventeen-year-old who had dialled 999, or the call handler.

'And where are you now?'

Liam did not hesitate.

'Linden Grove Country Park.'

'Is that a large place? Whereabouts are you in the park?'

'I'm at the Round Pond car park with a white Mini Clubman.'

'Is that your car?'

'It's my aunt's. Do you want the number plate?'

'Yes, please.'

Liam read the number. And then added helpfully: 'It's got L plates because she was teaching me to drive.'

'Where is your aunt now?'

'In the pond.'

The call handler did not miss a beat. They must be

trained not to react. I looked around the courtroom and the jury were certainly reacting. Their eyebrows were raised or they reorganized themselves in their seats or they simply froze in some unnatural position. They listened intently as, on request, Liam calmly gave his aunt's name and address.

'Please stay on the line until the emergency services arrive.'

'I'll wait by the car and then I can show them how to get to the pond,' said the ever-helpful Liam.

'Police and ambulance are on their way, someone should be with you in sixteen minutes.'

'Not much point in the ambulance, but thanks anyway, mate.'

The recording clicked off, the courtroom remained silent and the prosecution barrister paused for effect, studying his papers, before he looked across at me.

'Dr Harding, you are a consultant in both forensic psychiatry and child and adolescent psychiatry. You are recognized as an expert in your field. You have been the clinical lead for the Forensic Child and Adolescent Mental Health Services across a large part of London. Given your experience, would you say that the young man we have just heard was showing any indication of psychosis?'

'There is no overt evidence of psychosis.'

'Can you tell the court how you reach that conclusion?'

'If Liam had been psychotic, we might have expected his speech to be disorganized, resulting from disordered thinking. Changes in speech can be subtle, but the defence argues that Liam was acutely psychotic shortly before the recording we've heard. Psychotic to a degree that might explain him killing his aunt. In those circumstances I would expect to hear some evidence of psychosis in the recording.'

'So, his speech did not, in your opinion, indicate the disorder of psychosis?'

'Quite the opposite – his speech is clear and concise. His aunt has died but very shortly afterwards he is able to function mentally and converse over the phone. This is compelling evidence against the possibility that a few minutes earlier he had been acutely psychotic.'

'How might a psychotic person behave?'

'In a variety of ways. Sometimes psychosis can be overt – a person responding to hallucinations might have disordered speech and thought but they may also be overtly paranoid and suspicious. Or they might be fearful. Sometimes psychosis is more subtle, in which case there might be suspicion, confusion or delusional thoughts: things that are less evident in speech alone.'

The barrister nodded.

'Did you hear that in this recording?'

I shook my head. 'No. But this is about context, the context being that Liam's aunt had just been killed. Of course, I am also considering other material, such as body-worn video and the mental health assessment carried out soon after this call. If her killing had been substantially driven by psychosis, then I would expect there to be evidence of that psychosis, but I find no overt evidence of disordered speech or thought, suspiciousness or paranoia. For example, had Liam been paranoid, he might have withheld some of the information asked of him by the call handler.'

'And you find that he was not withholding?'

'He's not at all guarded. He appears to have thought ahead to the likely arrival of the police and is standing by the car to show them the way to the pond. He offers, without hesitation, his aunt's car number and he aids identification by adding that the car has L plates. He gives her name and address promptly without pausing. He thanks the operator for his help and, in a friendly and relaxed tone, then calls him "mate". His aunt has just been killed but in my view there is no sign of psychosis at all.'

Liam had strangled Miss Swinney and then pushed her in the pond. This was beyond doubt; he had readily admitted to the crime and the jury was not being asked to decide whether he was guilty or not guilty. No, this jury was choosing between manslaughter and murder.

The manslaughter verdict the defence wanted would mean that Liam had not intended to kill his aunt, that he had done so because he was mentally ill, substantially reducing his culpability. A manslaughter verdict would mean that the risk of Liam killing again was linked to his mental illness – so if his illness were treated, there would be a reduced risk of further violence. A manslaughter verdict would mean he would likely be treated in hospital and, once treated, be home within a few years and able to get on with life just as if he had not strangled a loved member of his family.

The defence psychiatrist was called Dr Graf. We had both interviewed Liam and come to different conclusions about him. Dr Graf was arguing that Liam had not meant to kill his aunt because he had been mentally ill, suffering from a temporary psychosis which diminished his responsibility for the crime. He had been arguing that all Wednesday and all Thursday.

Now it was Friday and I was on the witness stand for the prosecution.

'Dr Harding, the 999 recording was made at 1335 hours. We know that after killing Miss Swinney the defendant called the emergency services: he says the call was made less than ten minutes after his aunt's death. The forensic pathologist does agree with that timing. We have heard Dr Graf express the view that the defendant was psychotic at the time of the attack and that this was a temporary condition which passed.'

Yes, Dr Graf had expressed that view not just once but again and again under cross-examination, refusing to admit to any other possibility.

'If you do not think the defendant was psychotic when he called the emergency services, Dr Harding, might he have been psychotic ten minutes earlier when Miss Swinney was attacked?'

To answer the question, I turned to the jury. A mentor had told me years ago to make sure my feet always pointed at the jury and I had followed this advice all through my career.

'Psychosis that might account for such an expression of violence . . . ? Well, in my view that degree of psychosis would be unlikely to disappear within ten minutes.'

'You do not believe that even the transient psychosis that Dr Graf has diagnosed would disappear within ten minutes?'

'No.'

I glanced at Liam, as I had throughout his trial. He looked young, pale and withdrawn. Outside it was a grey, blustery winter's day. The school holidays had not finished and his mates were probably hanging around each other's houses or they were off skiing with their families – Liam had attended a very exclusive school. Now he sat, friendless, in a room with no windows. His head was bowed and between him and the court was a thick Perspex wall. His family was seated nearby but Liam didn't look at anyone. Occasionally, it was possible to see that he was crying because his shoulders were shaking. But mostly he was very, very still. He was a statue. He did not look up. He did not catch anyone's eye.

The prosecution barrister said: 'The defendant's mother and then his father spoke to him on Miss Swinney's phone about an hour before her death and neither reports any unusual, disordered or paranoid behaviour during the call. So if the defendant was psychotic, the disorder must have come and gone within one hour and ten minutes. Is that possible?'

'That would be highly unlikely. Psychosis doesn't just blow over, like, say . . .' I paused and spoke clearly. '. . . a temper tantrum. It is a serious condition, usually treated with medication. And, even with the right medication and support, there almost certainly could not be, in my view, in such a short time, a transformation from the disorder of psychosis to the ordered thinking we have just heard.'

'Are you aware that the defendant had any history of psychosis?'

'According to his medical records, he had none.'

'So he had never in the past been prescribed anti-psychotic medication?'

'No.'

'And you regard the recording of the defendant's 999 call as evidence that he was not psychotic?'

'Yes, I do. I should also draw your attention to the comments of the assessor who saw the defendant soon after he was arrested and taken to prison. She is highly trained to detect any sign of disordered thinking, inappropriate behaviour or paranoid delusion which might indicate psychosis. She found no such symptoms. In fact, she noted that he was the very opposite of psychotic: polite, coherent and responsive.'

'So, on his arrival at the prison, the defendant was not given medication for the temporary psychosis that Dr Graf has referred to?'

'No, because psychosis has never been diagnosed by anyone but Dr Graf.'

Touché, Dr Graf. I remained standing until mid-afternoon, when the court broke for the weekend. But, before we left, the judge commented that he wanted to know – and said he was sure the jury must want to know – why, if he was not psychotic, Liam had killed Miss Swinney? Out of the blue, for no apparent reason? And his victim was not a stranger but an aunt he had loved, a woman who had played a significant, generous role in his upbringing and to whom he would often turn in times of trouble.

The whole courtroom – the barristers in their wigs, the judge, the journalists tapping at their laptops, the public in the gallery, Liam's family crushing tissues in their hands, the straight-backed court clerks, everyone in that room wanted to know: why? Why had a boy done this terrible thing if he had not been insane at the time? There was only one person present who knew the answer, of course. And he wasn't saying.

2

Of course, I'd thought a lot about why Liam had killed his aunt. After years in general psychiatry, then focusing on the criminal mind in forensic psychiatry, and finally specializing in child and adolescent forensic psychiatry, I certainly had an idea about what may have happened between the aunt and her nephew that day. I suspected that the attack was the result of many complex emotions and one of those emotions was anger: my reference to a temper tantrum had not been casual.

Liam's parents ran their own business. They imported and marketed a luxury brand of women's shoes and their years of hard work had built both success and wealth. Their lives had been about heels, laces, soles and uppers, all of which left little time for Liam. He was an only child with busy parents but he had not been ignored: single and childless, his father's sister, Auntie Joy, had stepped up. Liam had spent as much time with her as with his parents.

He had always misbehaved at school. His career there had been notable for threats of violence, inappropriate behaviour, particularly around girls when he became a teenager, and bullying. At the time of the homicide, he was facing retakes after doing badly in his GCSEs. However, he had shown no sign of working for his exams. His parents had therefore chosen a drastic course of action.

They confiscated his phone.

This would be difficult for almost anyone, especially a teenager. Liam reacted with extreme fury. After a loud and long row with his parents, he called his aunt, who lived nearby, and said he wanted to visit her. His parents agreed to this. Liam strongly suspected that his parents had passed his mobile to Miss Swinney, and in fact he was right. She had been told to reward him with a few hours of phone time if he completed his schoolwork. Evidently, she had agreed to this. She, too, wanted Liam to concentrate and do well in his exams.

But Miss Swinney preferred the carrot to the stick. She was withholding Liam's phone as promised, but she had also told him that she would buy him a car if he passed all his GCSE retakes. So that day, when he showed no sign of studying, she would not give him his phone. Instead she had offered him driving practice. There had been a few lessons already, but he wanted more practice.

Liam drove them to Round Pond, a local and often deserted beauty spot. On arrival at the country park, he and Miss Swinney walked down to the pond. When they reached the pond, Liam used a dog lead to strangle his aunt.

Before the trial, I had met Liam at his secure unit. We discussed his relationship with his aunt. He told me how close they had been and how sad her death made him – as if he was not responsible for it. I asked him to tell me about that day with his aunt prior to her death and he said that she had been very angry with him for failing to study.

'She said she wanted to kill me. She stood in the kitchen saying she was going to take the lead she charged her phone with and wrap it around my neck and strangle me. She just stood there and said it! She really wanted to kill me.'

'You felt she was threatening you?'

'Yes!'

'Did you have an argument?'

'No. I was too scared.'

'Were you ever scared of your aunt before?'

'No, because she never said she wanted to kill me before. She took the phone charger and waved it at me. At my neck.'

So, was this a complex hallucinatory experience? Was it a delusion – a misplaced belief held with absolute conviction? Or maybe he had elaborated the facts to consolidate a sense of fear that he had truly experienced?

To reach the truth, I had to analyse not just what Liam said, but the way that he said it. The verbal and non-verbal cues, his physical presence in the room, his fear or lack of fear at recalling horror. And, in my opinion, Liam was not terrified. His recollection held no fear. He was even glib.

As for Miss Swinney, she worked at a senior level in human resources for a large company. I had read the character reports. It was hard to believe that she had made these threats and indeed Liam had not mentioned them to the police or to Dr Graf or any other professional. So this new description of events seemed to have been dropped into his narrative just for me. And, in my opinion, having seen many hundreds of cases over the years, it was fiction.

'So,' I continued, 'your aunt said she wanted to kill you . . . and then she offered to take you for a driving lesson?'

I wondered if this would sound as unbelievable to the jury as it did to me.

'Yeah. Then when we got to the pond, she said she was going to drown me.'

'Whose idea was it to go to Round Pond?'

'Hers. She said it was to give me driving practice, but when we got to the pond, she said she wanted to push me in and kill me. I was scared.'

'Did you ask for your phone back when you got to the country park?'

'Yeah. So I could take some pictures of the pond.'

'But she didn't give it to you?'

'She said she didn't have it.'

But the phone had been there and Liam must have known it, because he had used it to call 999. I asked him to tell me how he had recovered it, to tell me more about that day, but he said he couldn't remember anything else. Nothing. No memory of any anger or row. No memory of walking to the pond's edge from the car. No memory of strangling Miss Swinney or pushing her into the water.

I had visited the pond and found it surrounded by trees and shrubs. There were very few places where you could easily push someone in, and still fewer where you could do so from any height. It seemed to me that the spot must have been chosen in advance and it was more likely to have been chosen by Liam than his aunt.

'Why was there a dog lead? I understand your Auntie Joy didn't have a dog.'

'She kept it in the car because she walked the neighbours' dog sometimes.'

'But why did you carry it with you to the pond?'

'Auntie carried it down there. When we got to the pond, she said she wanted to push me in. And she had the dog lead and I remembered how she had waved the phone charger around and talked about strangling me and I thought she was going to strangle me with the dog lead.'

'So you had to wrestle it away from her?'

He shrugged and looked down. He had a thin face and had evidently been working out in the secure unit's gym, so that his head looked strangely small on his developed upper body.

I asked: 'Why do you think you pushed her in the water after strangling her? The pathologist said she was dead, you could have just left her.'

Once again, Liam shrugged helplessly as though he hadn't been there at all by the pond that day.

'If you remember so little, did you ever think someone else might have done this?'

Of course, the absence of DNA evidence meant the police had ruled out third party involvement. But I was interested in Liam's answer.

He did not hesitate. 'I knew it must have been me. Because no one else was there.'

My own theory was that Liam, as driver, albeit a learner, had held on to the car keys. This would have given him some power in that lonely place. I thought he had asked his aunt for his phone and she had refused to give it back. I don't know if he threatened her. But I daresay she did not think it possible that her beloved nephew, a boy who was almost a son to her, would produce the dog lead and wrap it around her neck. The pathologist had learned from the ligature marks that her assailant had stood in front of her as she died and so would have seen her eyes bulge and her skin turn purple. A steely determination to kill is required to watch that and not loosen the ligature.

I feared that Liam had planned the attack, chosen his weapon and selected the pondside location so that he could be sure his aunt would die by drowning if he failed to kill her by strangling her. Or maybe he had planned to drown her and only thought of strangling her when he saw the dog lead in the car.

I did not believe his action had been caused by psychosis: finding that place by the pond where you could push someone in, taking the dog lead; it all required ordered pre-planning. And psychosis is a condition of disorganization. As an expert witness I had to examine the facts and present my evidence impartially and clearly for the jury so that they could make a decision. No matter how adversarial the courtroom felt, I reminded myself as a witness to remain neutral. But as a human, of course I had fears and instincts. And mine told me that Liam was a very dangerous young man.

A lot rested on the jury's verdict. Manslaughter should take him to hospital, where he would be treated for mental illness and probably assumed to be safe after treatment and a relatively short stay. A jail sentence for murder would be longer and in jail he would ideally undergo psychological offender programmes to reduce his risk. Hospital might seem a more compassionate place for him to be, but it could only reduce risk if he was mentally ill.

The case had taken a long time to come to trial and he was now eighteen. The press was therefore allowed to report from the courtroom – and the journalists were relishing it. Miss Swinney's death after the driving lesson was enough for them to dub the defendant Killer Learner Liam.

The jury was shown out that Friday and we all rose for the judge's exit and then there was a brief pause as everyone transited from hushed courtroom mode to the demands of everyday life. The barristers gathered their papers, the police picked up their laptops, people in the gallery stretched and stood up and switched on their phones, journalists chattered as they stuffed equipment into their bags. I could not talk to the police or the prosecution barrister or anyone at all about the case because I was part-way through giving my evidence. I felt oddly isolated after standing alone in the witness box all day. No one spoke to me, no one looked at me.

I packed my books and reports into my bag, glimpsing Dr Graf from the corner of my eye as he slipped away. Then I stepped down from the box.

Still feeling exposed, I left the courtroom. And walked straight into Liam's family, who were standing in a huddle in the corridor. A few of them glared at me; others dropped their voices significantly at the sight of a prosecution witness. His parents simply looked away.

For the first time, I wondered what they were really thinking about Liam. Secretly. Maybe they had fears about him that they could not even voice to each other. They must have been well aware of the many incidents of his violent behaviour at school. Perhaps his parents believed, as I did, that Liam was dangerous. They would have to live alongside that knowledge while they grieved for his victim. And the knowledge that, if he could watch horror and pain on the face of a loved aunt as he killed her, then he was, perhaps, capable of killing any one of them. But at the same time, he was their son. They loved him.

As I got on the train to go home, yet again I reflected on how hard it was to be a parent; how hard it would be for me.

3

It was my first day at school. My mother took me to the gate. Crutches forward, click. Swish, as she swung her paralysed legs between them, her skirt fluttering. Donk. As her heavy boots, stabilized by callipers, landed on the ground ahead, taking her weight for just a moment while she moved her crutches forward again. Click, her crutches hitting the ground. Swish, her skirt. Donk, her boots. Click. Swish. Donk. As familiar and loved a rhythm as my own heartbeat.

The rhythm stopped at the gates. My heart, however, beat on. Hard and fast. I felt so sick that I barely noticed the other kids staring at her.

At break time, a big boy loomed over me.

'Your mum,' he said knowledgeably, 'is a spaz.'

I didn't know what a spaz was, but it sounded as though it could be something out of *Dr Who* and I loved Dr Who. He was kind and good and fair. I hoped the spaz was an ally of the Doctor. I nodded wisely. Yes, my mother probably was a spaz.

Some other children arrived and stood very close. I wanted to move back but there were more children standing behind me.

'His mum's a spastic! His mum's a spastic!' they chanted.

'What's a spastic?' I asked my mother that evening, when we'd donked, clicked and swished our way home, the sickness in my stomach entirely gone now, replaced by hunger.

She was making tea, her elbows leaning on her crutches. She rolled her eyes.

'Take no notice,' she said.

'But what does it mean?'

She shook her head and pursed her lips.

'Marching time. Come on. March the knives and forks over to the table, will you? Then be a good soldier, march back again and carry the veg through.'

I did a lot of marching. Every mealtime, and whenever my mother had washing to haul into the machine or was trying to hang it out, or if she was brushing the kitchen floor or doing anything really, I marched. I was a good soldier who did what she could not: anything requiring two hands (click) and two legs (swish).

Dad was out at the pub so it was quiet at home tonight. After tea, my mother and I sat in front of the fire. As a special treat, we turned on three bars and my knees roasted pleasantly. I told her about school and how I had already started learning to read. She nodded approval.

'It is very important,' Mum said, 'to be a good reader and learn as much as you can. That way you will get a good job.'

I watched as she lit a cigarette. She always had a packet in her pocket and, when she sat down, it made a soft, crinkling sound.

'Did you get a good job?' I asked.

Mum breathed out smoke and looked embarrassed. 'I never should have been sent away to that horrible school for kids in wheelchairs. I certainly wasn't going to hang around there and take exams.'

'Would you have passed them?'

'Oh, I daresay I would have. But I did typing instead.'

'Where?'

'London. I was just sixteen and I set off for London with next to nothing and no job, just a lot of . . .' She paused. Her face suddenly looked girlish, ringed by blond hair, her eyes big as though she longed for something.

'A lot of what? Money?' I asked.

'Not money. Just a lot of hope in my heart.'

I imagined Mum, her shrunken legs inside their metal frames, her great black boots dangling from them, doing donk, click, swish all the way to London, which I knew to be far, far away from the north of England. Mum, going all that way, with hope in her heart.

'Did you go by yourself?'

'I did. I nearly broke your grandad's heart.'

I loved my grandfather very much. He was kind and good and fair, like Dr Who, and he had given me my very own Dr Who. The silent figure stood on the mantelpiece now, watching over me, the way Grandad watched over me when he visited. I tried to imagine Grandad's heart breaking. Grandad crying, because Mum had gone to London. It made me want to cry, too.

'What happened when you got there?' I asked.

'I found the Swinging Sixties, a place to live, took a job and met your father.' She glanced at me. 'The Swinging Sixties is just an expression – there weren't any swings, love. They were years when everyone had fun.'

‘What sort of fun?’

‘Singing and dancing.’

‘Did you have fun?’ I knew my mother sang very nicely but I could not imagine her dancing, not with her crutches.

Her eyes were big now. She was remembering all the hope in her heart.

‘Oh yes,’ she said softly.

And at that moment, I knew what I was going to do when I grew up. I was going to put hope in Mum’s heart by becoming a doctor. Like Dr Who. I would be a doctor who was kind and good and fair. And I would cure her polio so that she could dance.

Many years later, when I was taking A-levels, I explained to the school’s careers advisor that I wanted to study medicine. I didn’t mention Dr Who, of course, but I probably told her about Mum’s polio.

She looked at me very hard and then shook her head.

‘I think we should be realistic, Duncan.’

‘Really, that’s what I’m going to do.’

‘I don’t think so.’

‘But –’

‘Duncan, no one from this school has ever reached university.’

I glanced out of the window. It was raining. Grey houses in long rows. Their roofs were wet but not shining.

She said: ‘I mean, you might be the first; it’s just possible you could get in to study a science subject. But medicine requires very high grades.’

‘I can work for those grades!’

The teacher had bobbed blond hair and now she looked

at me sadly and shook her head again, so vigorously this time that her hair swished from side to side.

'You're just going to be disappointed if you carry on like this. Have you thought of working in a laboratory? You can be a lab technician if your A-levels are good enough.'

A few weeks later, that same teacher came to a gig. Ever since I was fourteen, I'd been playing guitar and singing. All through my teenage years I'd formed and reformed bands, and this band was good. We played the school gig to a wildly enthusiastic audience.

The teacher wrote me a letter.

Duncan, after this evening I am left in no doubt about where your future lies. Keep going with that music, you have real talent: other unrealistic aspirations can only get in your way.

I knew she meant well. And of course I'd thought of becoming a musician. But the letter had unintended consequences. It helped me to find something in myself that I had seen in my mother so many times. Since we had sat at the fireside and she had told me about having hope in her heart, she had studied for O-levels, A-levels, a degree. Now she had a good job in a museum. Her journey had not been easy, but she had done it. Whenever people looked at Mum on her crutches and thought she couldn't do something, she was absolutely sure to do it. I re-read the teacher's letter and I knew one thing for certain. I was going to be a doctor.

When I went to medical school in London there was a point in the first few weeks when I decided the careers advisor had been right. I should stop all this, go back up north, where people spoke like me, and become a musician. London was overwhelming in its noise, its vastness, its great indifference. And the other medical students, many from private schools and almost all middle-class, were overwhelming in their confidence.

Even the course was overwhelming: not because I found the work hard but because I had misunderstood the prospectus. I had not realized that dissecting a cadaver meant cutting up a human body. I had assumed that a cadaver was some sort of reptile, a lizard perhaps. The greyness of the long-dead human body, the smell of formaldehyde, the cold weight of the scalpel, the echo of the tiled labs: it was literally the stuff of nightmares. I thought only of home. Until slowly, surely, fascination quashed horror and London's buzz became the buzz of life itself.

Academically I did well, so well that an opportunity came up for me to take a break halfway through my medical training and move into research. I grabbed it.

My subject: polio, of course. Specifically, the motor neurons, those nerve cells that for so many years had stubbornly refused to convey their single message – 'Move!' – to my mother's leg muscles.

I studied the neuro-muscular junction, the point where the message should be passed to her muscles but wasn't. Thanks to vaccines, there were no recent cases of polio in the UK, but as earlier victims reached late middle age, many were giving way to post-polio syndrome. Polio's last shout. This was the subject of my research, ostensibly. But secretly, I had not given up my boyhood vow to cure my mother's polio. And my mother had not given up hope that I would do just that. I could not forget that private, hidden place I occasionally visited inside my head, where my mother got up and danced without support. Or walked across a room. Down a street. Along a beach. Mum, striding out. No crutches. No callipers. No sniggers of laughter behind her. No staring kids. No nasty jokes. Just a woman walking.

Research turned out to be a cruel master. It is almost entirely dependent on commercial funding and no one was interested in funding polio research since it had now become a disease of the developing world. My work was proving useful for other motor neuron diseases, but it wasn't helping my mother. It took years to understand that it couldn't. It was simply impossible to replace a missing neuro-muscular junction.

I finally had to accept that I could do nothing about my mother's polio. When I told her, she was furious. Her faith in me had been absolute. She believed that if anyone could get her walking, that person would be her clever son. And when he told her that he could not, she felt betrayed. And angry. Very angry.

She did not speak to me for a year and her reaction helped me to understand something I had always known, even as a child, even as a medical student learning about every aspect of the human body. That mental health is just as important for a patient's welfare as physical health. Even though her polio was incurable, even though it was a physical condition, living with it had greatly affected her mental well-being. Someone should have given my mother mental health support long ago.

Eventually I had to stop neurological research and finish my medical studies. I had diverted for so many years that now I had to qualify or give up my dream of becoming a doctor. So I returned to the study of clinical medicine and found myself embracing it. Each specialism was exciting, each patient so fascinating that most are still imprinted indelibly on my mind today. And it is just possible that the eleven years it took me to finish medical school broke some kind of record.

Here I was in 2001, aged thirty, a doctor at last. But after a brief period of excitement and pride, I had begun to hate it. There were many wards and many hospitals. Bodies lay haemorrhaging blood and other fluids while their owners looked at me for help that no one could give. Patients died before my eyes; others suffered agonies no painkiller could relieve. There wasn't a war on. It was a normal day. Other people go into medicine for exactly this, but I realized now that it was exactly this that I had detoured into research to avoid.

Finally a train crash, the resulting chaos at the hospital, a night of trauma and too many tragedies told me I should take time out to think. I worked as a musician for a few years, funding myself with locum shifts and busking (I earned more busking) while I asked myself: what sort of doctor did I want to be?

After all those years of research into motor neurons, neurology was the obvious answer. But neurology was tainted for me by my failure to cure my mother's polio or help it at all. I did not want to be a neurologist. What, then?

The answer appeared one day on a locum shift. And when it came, it was so obvious that I wondered if it had been shouting at me all along but I had chosen not to hear.

It was a hot day in summer. A slight breeze outside. Pollen resting in the air along with exhaust fumes.

The old hospital had various courtyards and gardens and for most of the year they were too cool, damp and shady for patients. But on a day like this, all the courtyard doors were open. I had an unpleasant task ahead of me. To walk through one of those doors and find an elderly woman in order to tell her that she was now a widow.

I had met her earlier. She had said that today was her diamond wedding anniversary: she had married the patient exactly sixty years ago. And now I had to inform her that in future this date would mark a different anniversary.

'It's all right,' she said, as I approached her shady bench. 'I know.'

I stared at her and hesitated.

'I can tell from your face. You didn't really want to come out here and say it to me, did you? But it's all right, love. I know you all did your best. His time was up.'

'It was very peaceful, Mrs Hegarty. He just slipped away from us.'

'That's him, that's Ernie all over. No fuss. Don't suppose you smoke?'

I shook my head. Of course, I greatly disapproved of smoking and had even recently persuaded my mother to give up.

'Mind if I do?'

Yes. But in the circumstances I assured her that the answer was no.

She lit a match, deftly, with one hand, a move which requires so much practice that it is usually the sign of an accomplished, long-term smoker.

'See,' she said, 'this is what we did together. We smoked. We knew each other so well that we hardly had to talk. We sat smoking and we just knew what the other one was thinking. And you won't believe it but I sat on this bench with a cigarette and it made me feel so close to him, as if we were sitting here together. So don't you tell me smoking's bad for me, Doctor.'

I smiled. 'What about that day you married, sixty years ago? Was it hot like this?'

There was a strange, cackling, smoke-filled sound. A sort of laugh.

'Nothing like today! It poured with rain and my mother shook her head and said: hmmm, that's not a good sign, I'm not sure you'll have a long and happy marriage to Ernie!' She cackled again. 'He was such a quiet, thoughtful young fellow and she wasn't used to that. She couldn't understand a man who didn't bash her.'

I encouraged her to talk more about Ernie and their life together. It had been hard and they had been very poor, but they had clearly been bound by something deeper than their vows. I envied their children. I could not imagine having two parents who loved each other.

We sat talking until a nurse came to call me in.

'We've been looking everywhere for you,' she scolded as we made our way back into the building.

'I was telling Mrs Hegarty that Mr Hegarty had died.'

'But how long does that take!' she demanded. It was not really a question.

So, how long should it take? How much time should you spend with someone at such a major and emotional turning point in her life? Apparently, no time at all if you worked in a busy NHS hospital. The nurse continued: 'The ward's bursting at the seams and we need you to sign off four patients because A&E have at least six waiting to come in. One is an attempted suicide and, good gracious, just wait until you see her wrists.'

My mother threatened suicide frequently. She was strong and determined but, starting from my primary school days, had often warned me as I set off with my school bag that she might kill herself today. I seldom returned home without bracing myself to find her dead body. Now I was thirty and her threats still filled me with anxiety and sent me rushing north when she phoned. As a child I could do nothing but remain very quiet in the face of her misery. But now, as a doctor, I thought the best thing to do with someone who was suicidal was talk to them.

I wondered how much time I could spend with the patient with the spectacularly cut wrists. One glance at the nurse, her jaw set, her hands clenched, answered that. She was under pressure and angry with the doctor for wasting time. There was no way I would be allowed to sit and talk to patients today or ever. I would have to treat them with medication and move rapidly to the next.

And so the ward patients became again an endless conveyor belt. See them, treat them, move them on, see more, treat them, move them on . . .

That locum shift pointed me in the direction my life and career should take. I knew that I wanted to spend time with patients. I wanted to listen to them. I wanted them to talk about themselves. I wanted to help them lead more hopeful, happier lives, because I understood that mental health is as important as physical health. In fact, I wanted to be a psychiatrist. Obviously!

4

I won a coveted trainee place at London's, perhaps the UK's, leading psychiatric hospital. I was immediately caught up in a maelstrom of patients who had many different ways of perceiving and interpreting the world. Back on my locum shift, I had wanted to stop and talk to the suicidal. Well, here they were, in this huge and bustling hospital, each one with their own needs and complexities.

Early on I met Gregory. I heard about him first on a ward round, soon after he had been detained in the hospital against his will.

'Acutely suicidal,' said the consultant. 'Damn nearly succeeded in killing himself. And obviously psychotic. Keeps going on about being on television because of some sort of catastrophic business disaster. The usual stuff. Claims it affected hundreds of people, says it led to relationship failure. Not actually insisting Beyoncé was his partner, but I wouldn't be surprised if he does. Says this colossal failure, as shown on TV, was all his fault, et cetera, et cetera.'

We nodded wisely. Clearly, the man was psychotic.

Psychosis is a disconnection from reality. If a layman dials 999 and says someone has gone mad, it generally means the patient is psychotic. This may take many different forms – hearing voices, seeing things, delusions, believing in some alternative reality. And it is commonplace for the psychotic to talk big. TV fame. Immense events involving celebrities or leading politicians. Overuse of words like catastrophic and colossal. Yep. We'd heard it all before. Gregory was surely psychotic.

Then I met him and recognized him at once.

'Er . . . it's all true,' I told the consultant.

He looked horrified.

'There really was a TV programme about him: I know because I saw it. He had a huge shipping company and two ships went down, some crew lost their lives, the shares plummeted and loads of people were made redundant, questions were asked in Parliament and I think there was a lot of talk about negligence and corporate manslaughter . . .'

The consultant raised his eyebrows. The rest of the team looked at each other. We weren't used to big talk being true around here.

This was a game changer, because now the question we had to ask ourselves was: if Gregory was not psychotic but simply showing a rational reaction to a real-life catastrophe, did we have any right to detain him here against his will? If he was able to make a decision, based on rational and sound reasoning, to take his own life, should we interfere? Or just let him kill himself?

Of course, as doctors, we wanted to prolong life. But we also had to respect a patient's wishes and if a rational patient wanted to die, who were we to stop him by keeping him here under lock and key? I personally find it very difficult and upsetting to deprive anyone of their liberty. But at the same time, I could see how great Gregory's suffering was and I really wanted us to continue to care for him.

It was a fine line to walk, but eventually we decided that it was right to keep him in the hospital, even though he protested. We knew there was a good chance that, if we could support Gregory through this acute period of suicidal impulse, using the twin psychiatric weapons of medication and empathic communication, the need to kill himself might pass. This was true of many other, even more obviously ill patients. By detaining them, we aimed to get them through the worst and release them with at least a sense of hope. After that, there was follow-up treatment in the community to help them approach their problems more holistically. If they chose to, they might come to understand their own psyche and recognize what part of themselves they wished to annihilate. And why. And whether there was an alternative to annihilation.

So Gregory stayed on the ward. He was furious. At first, there was no change. Days passed and he remained withdrawn, evidently without hope and intent on committing suicide the moment we released him. Days turned to weeks. How long could we do this for? We debated this, aware of the long line of patients waiting for admittance.

And then he began, very slowly, to strengthen. His desperate need to kill himself became gradually less intense while we talked to him a lot and treated him for depression, not psychosis. Eventually, when he had regained a sense of hope for the future, he was discharged into the care of the community mental health team. We had locked him up against his will. And saved his life.

There are many ways of killing yourself and over the next few years I would learn that the suicidal can be very inventive. Anyone who had tried and failed to die went first to A&E. They had to be cleared medically before we could admit them to a psychiatric ward. Whatever physical harm they had done – damaged their heart, stomach or neck, inflicted wounds, burns or fractures – had to be treated first.

'Hello, Petra,' I began, visiting a patient who was waiting in a side room off A&E for clearance to join the psychiatric ward. 'I'm Dr Harding. Tell me what happened to bring you here today.'

Petra was about fifty years old. Her hair had not been cut for a while: it hung, limp and grey, to her shoulders. She had chiselled features which might have once been very fine but were now so asymmetrical that she looked like a young child's drawing.

She did not meet my eye, but I watched her facial expression. It was one I was learning to recognize very quickly in the psychotic. Not so much confused as perplexed. A sort of bewilderment which seemed to say that the world did not really make sense. A patient could tell you absolutely nothing but reveal they were psychotic from this strange, dazed look alone.

Petra did not respond to me at all. In fact, although she did not actually pull the bed covers up over her face, metaphorically she certainly did. I doubted that I would get a word out of this shut-down woman.

'I've been looking at your notes. It seems that you tried to fill a room with car exhaust?'

Silence. According to the notes, Petra had run a hose from a car outside her window into her house.

'Carbon monoxide can give you a terrible headache; I hope you're feeling better now?'

Silence.

'Your notes say that you have a diagnosis of bipolar affective disorder, Petra, so I suppose you must have reached a very low point. That makes me wonder if we've got your medication right. I'm hoping you'll agree to be admitted to our psychiatric ward and then we can try to adjust your pills so they work better for you. Maybe you'd like to talk about how you've been feeling, too?'

Medication is very difficult to prescribe for bipolar affective disorder because, by definition, the patient swings between the highs of mania and perhaps euphoria down to the deep, deep lows of depression. Of course, anti-depressants can help as the patient plunges downwards. But, as the pendulum moves the other way, that same medication can push patients faster and higher into a dangerous state of mania.

And now Petra spoke. She still did not look at me but she said, very firmly: 'No.'

'You don't want to change your medication?'

'I want to go home.'

'Petra, I think it would be good to take care of you for a while.'

'No, no, I want to go home, I have to go, I must go home.' Her voice was flat, almost expressionless. But I could hear the steel in it.

I tried to sound reasonable. 'Nothing's changed though, has it? You feel the same way you felt when you tried to kill yourself. So what are the chances you'll try again?'

At first, she did not reply but studied, with that same, distant, perplexed expression, the hospital blanket that lay across her. Finally she said: 'I want to die. You've no right to stop me.'

I sighed. We were stepping into the fog together.

'Wouldn't it be wise to spend time with us?' I heard my

own voice. Kind. Reasonable. 'At least so that we can discuss all this?'

'No.'

If we released her, she would try again to kill herself, I had no doubt of that. But was she correct that I had no right to stop her? Actually, I did have that right, if I thought the patient was not sound and rational enough to make such an important decision. And, since I believed she was psychotic, I was sure that her decision to die could not be a rational one.

I consulted colleagues and they agreed with me. So, with many doubts, worries and misgivings, Petra became the first patient I Sectioned. That meant I was detaining her under Section 2 of the Mental Health Act. Three mental health professionals, two of them doctors, must give their consent for this – if they agree that it is necessary to detain the patient for their own safety or that of others.

I felt truly terrible, locking up Petra on a ward against her will.

'Jailer!' she hissed, her asymmetrical face twisting her features into strange hieroglyphics that spelled hatred.

But over the next few days, psychosis left her, the depression eased and she grew more open and relaxed. I made sure I spent as much time with her as possible and she chatted happily to me. She enjoyed this and, since I was busy, I asked if the ward psychologist might be available for further work with her. I had already found working with psychologists rewarding: our combined skills could be highly effective in treating patients.

I should say that only psychiatrists are medical doctors who can prescribe medication. Psychologists are not usually qualified to diagnose illness or medicate in the same way. However, they might often view a patient broadly and holistically and, participating in a treatment plan, undertake very useful therapeutic work. Just what Petra needed. But unfortunately no psychologist was available.

My own approach, wherever possible, involved working with patients in a psychological way, so I decided to make as much time as possible to continue my talks with Petra.

She told me that she had grown up in a large house in Richmond with every comfort – but that there had been some difficult parental behaviour. We concluded together that neither parent had psychotic episodes, but that both had suffered from deep depression.

'When were you first diagnosed?' I asked her.

'I had a few wobbles in my late twenties but really it first happened when I was about your age. I was thirty-two. I haven't worked since then.'

Petra lived in sheltered housing, where there was a warden: it was the warden who had heard the car engine and discovered the hose before the carbon monoxide had taken its toll.

'What job did you do?'

'I was deputy editor of a magazine.'

She named a well-known women's publication, famous for showing top models wearing eye-wateringly expensive clothes. I tried to imagine a younger Petra going off to work each day, her hair cut fashionably, her face expertly made up. She told me how she had commissioned articles and photographers and named some of the celebrities she had personally interviewed. There was enough information to convince me this was true. It was hard to associate the woman she had been before with the Petra I knew. Her mental illness had robbed her of so much. And it was chronic. It could not be cured. That was the reason she wanted to die.

We got on well, but there was a fundamental difference between us.

Petra wanted to go home to kill herself. I wanted her to stay. And I hoped to stabilize her here so that she might wish to live. I was aware that the danger for her would be compounded, or anyway changed, as her depression turned to mania. Once manic, she would engage in different behaviours but they would be just as risky. I really did not want her to leave until she felt safe and saw that life was not such a bleak place without hope. Even though a rational part of me asked just who I was to decide when life was tolerable, I ignored that voice.

I explained to Petra all the risks I wanted to protect her from. She nodded as if she agreed – but then appealed to the mental health tribunal to overrule me and release her.

The tribunal is independent. The three members interview everyone involved – patient, doctors, nurses, maybe relatives – and then decide whether to overrule the medics and release the patient. The tribunal is very like a court and it is the detailed, focused mechanism which is surely required when someone is locked up against their will.

What bad luck that my first Section and my first mental health tribunal were the same case. I had hated locking up Petra. And now I hated arguing for her enforced stay. But I believed that she should be detained for her own safety. I pleaded passionately with the tribunal, so passionately that I must have sounded inexperienced and naïve.

'Dr Harding wouldn't let me see a psychologist,' Petra

told the tribunal, throwing me narrow-eyed glances. 'I like talking to psychologists. But he just wanted to treat me himself.'

Not true really, but, yes, I had wanted to treat Petra holistically, balancing her medication with more psychological needs: I was already finding that to be effective for other patients. But Petra's accusation hit home with the tribunal. They looked at me dispassionately. I think one of them might have shaken her head.

I had to ask myself why I was so involved with this case. There was something familiar about the very deep feelings it stirred. Because my mother had been threatening suicide since I was a child, I had grown up determined to save her at all costs. She may have a good job now, her own house, a social life. But she was still capable of phoning me in the morning to inform me that she might very well choose to die by lunchtime. And of course I would always rush to save her. So now, was I simply trying to do the same for Petra?

I tried to stay detached and professional, but I could see that Petra was already moving out of depression and into a more manic phase of her illness. She hardly slept and ran around the ward talking intensely to everyone, making ludicrous promises. In some patients, extreme generosity to others is a feature of their illness and with Petra it was about the things she would buy her new friends. The fun they would have together. The places they would go.

I was sure we should monitor her and try to protect her from this next, potentially dangerous mood swing.

The tribunal did not agree. Their scepticism infuriated me and I was foolish enough to show it. Frowning at me, they released her. As they gave their verdict, my face reddened with anger and disappointment. I did not feel the tribunal had heard me. I wanted to shout: 'This is a mistake!'

Petra, who had been present throughout, turned to me triumphantly. But I could see that she was angry too. Angry with me, angry with the arguments I had made for detaining her.

She was free now, and she went to gather her things. A distant relative had arrived to give evidence, a cousin she hardly knew and had not seen for many years. He had expressed strongly his view to the tribunal that she should not be locked up and they had listened to him. Now he watched over her while she threw her belongings into a bag. His arms were folded and his stance said that it was his job to protect her from overbearing doctors like me who wanted to be psychologists as well as psychiatrists and might wish to obstruct her exit.

'I can never forgive you,' Petra hissed at me on her way out with him, 'for the things you said about me to the tribunal.'

Two weeks later, she was back.

On release, she had rapidly reached her manic high and was now crashing down from it once more into a deep and destructive depression.

I soon learned what had happened. The cousin had left her at her doorstep and disappeared. Within a few days, Petra had fallen victim to overblown delusion. Being manic, feeling happy and elated and invulnerable, fired by her sense of destructive omnipotence, she had made disastrous financial decisions. She had spent a fortune. She had then leased an expensive car and finally entered into a finance deal with a digger company. I never established why she thought she needed the digger.

She was now very depressed and acutely suicidal, and this was compounded by her new financial reality. She was being chased, mercilessly, for money she had spent but did not have. With her permission, I explained the situation to her creditors and tried my hardest to persuade them to cancel the contracts. But the credit card and leasing companies would have none of it. She was stuck with horrific and unpayable debts, as well as an expensive new car and a huge digger that was accumulating parking fines.

One reason bipolar affective disorder is so hard to manage is that, when the patient is manic, they feel very well. Some patients claim that this is when they are at their happiest and most creative. Do they want this experience subdued by medication? Of course not. They want to forget the utter misery of the depression that preceded it and must surely follow. But, to keep patients stable, the illness must be managed when they are near a high rather than when they are plummeting downwards. Doctors must listen, because generally patients can recognize their own warning signs of an impending drop, even if they cannot do anything to stop it. That is the time for a doctor to step in.

We did not need to Section Petra now: she consented to stay. I am glad to say that we did succeed in stabilizing her before she was released. A psychologist was available this time, holding intensive therapy sessions, while I focused on balancing her medication. Best of all, her social worker took on the leasing companies and, after much hard effort, eventually persuaded them to take the car and digger away and back off.

I don't want to give the impression that Petra's story had a happy ending. Her problems were sorted out and she was stabilized but I have no way of knowing that this worked in the long term. I did not see her again. Either because she was never readmitted. Or because she finally made a successful suicide attempt.

From Petra and so many of the other patients I met on the acute wards, there was a terrible lesson to be learned. I had become a doctor to fix people. At first I had hoped to fix my mother's polio. When I had realized this was impossible, when I had found there were many other patients I could not fix physically, I had hoped anyway to fix people's mental health problems. And now, as a psychiatrist, I realized that I could very seldom do that either. A breakdown in mental health is not like a broken ankle. I began to wonder why I had not become an orthopaedic surgeon: most of their patients seemed to heal eventually. Petra was one of many psychiatric patients who suffered from chronic and enduring conditions which could never be fully cured. Her bipolar affective disorder was her constant companion and there was no way to rid her of it, only to help her manage it.

What could we realistically hope to achieve? I asked myself this sometimes as I dashed from patient to patient, into A&E, back to the wards and sometimes out into the community. But there was no time to think, only time to work. And soon I had a new job. It was essential to move around to different hospitals and different clinics to gain experience in sub-specialities. Now I was going somewhere entirely different. A children's clinic.

5

My mother had recently retired from the museum to a seaside village where she lived in an ill-advised fisherman's cottage. She loved its age and its character, but the fishermen who had lived there had of course been able-bodied and for her the house was a struggle. Not least because it was at the top of a steep hill. The whole village was hills. And so she had given in, after all those years of refusing to use a wheelchair, and bought a motorized mobility scooter.

She had taken it out just once. A carload of teenagers had stopped and shouted abuse, showering her with litter. She had not used the scooter since and had barely left the house.

'I'm thinking of moving down south,' she told me. 'Nearer you.'

Having her close would mean fewer emergency journeys to the far north of England whenever she fell over or became very sad. Perhaps, if she lived nearby, she would be happier. And looking after her would have less impact on my life and relationships than all the emergency dashes.

I mostly lived at a girlfriend's flat these days and so it was easy to offer my mother the small house I had bought in east London. She moved in just as I started my new job at the child developmental neuropsychiatry clinic.

It was run by an eminent professor and I was lucky to work with him. I didn't know much about children but I was pretty sure of one thing: they should not be medicated if at all possible. The professor, however, had become famous for his treatment of Attention Deficit Hyperactivity Disorder. And his treatment was medication. Specifically, stimulants.

I could not hide my scepticism. He listened carefully while I told him why I felt that giving amphetamine salts to children was a very dangerous game.

'It certainly is!' he agreed, to my surprise.

'And surely this stuff is over-prescribed,' I added.

'Yes,' he said, 'it is.'

I had not learned much at that stage about Attention Deficit Hyperactivity Disorder. I knew that kids with this condition can't sit still or concentrate. I also knew ADHD had only quite recently blown in from across the Atlantic. Like hysteria in the early twentieth century, it was one of those non-infectious health conditions that never seemed to have existed before it was diagnosed, and then suddenly it was everywhere.

In the USA, ADHD had famously become the go-to diagnosis for wealthy middle-class kids whose exam grades weren't what their parents hoped. A dose of amphetamines could work wonders for low- or under-achievers: all a doctor had to do was diagnose ADHD and the amphetamine salts could produce satisfying results. And, since these amphetamines can allegedly boost the grades of just about everyone, there was soon a black market for them among university students, among anyone, in fact, facing an exam.

Now the UK was following exactly the same pattern. Private ADHD clinics were mushrooming everywhere so that the wealthy could get their kids a prescription for better exam results.

And here I was in a clinic, albeit an NHS one, which specialized in this fashionable condition.

'It is concerning,' the professor agreed, 'Ritalin and Adderall, for instance, are definitely over-prescribed. But that doesn't mean every prescription's wrong. I'm going to arrange for you to see a patient.'

'Are they coming into the clinic?'

'Yes, but before that you should pay a school visit. I'd like you to see how a normal day looks for Benjamin.'

Benjamin's school proved to be not far from where I lived. I had even noticed the place. It was one of London's old, redbrick primary schools with metal staircases running up the outside walls. It might once have seemed a grim building but now the small playground was painted in many colours and there were bright pictures stuck on the windows.

I arrived at break time and the yard, behind its security fence, was thick with pupils. They ran and played at density in what space was available. The receptionist buzzed me in and I threaded my way carefully through the tight knots of racing children.

'Dr Harding? So you've come to see our Benjamin!' said the receptionist, smiling with a certain significance.

'You know him?'

'Oh, everyone knows Benjamin.'

She led me to a classroom where the teacher was busy setting up the next lesson. I entered and felt sick. The smell of the place, the squeak of shoes on school flooring, the sight of groups of small tables with a maths puzzle on each one, the named workbooks, the pots of pens . . . briefly I returned to the misery of my own school years. Had I spent a single day at primary school without kids laughing at my mother or bullying me?

'I understand that you're working with the professor and he sent you to see Benjamin in class?' the teacher said.

I nodded. Outside, bells were ringing and whistles blowing, and the children were lining up to come in.

'I know he's going for treatment soon and all I can say to you is: let's hope it works and thank you, thank you, thank you.'

Well, now I was very curious. What was it about Benjamin?

The teaching assistant led the class in. They were eight- and nine-year-olds. They arrived in a line. Some were talking, some were looking around. In places the line was ragged. A few kids rushed towards their workbooks, others ambled here and there looking for their places before sitting down. Just one child was different. He did not walk into the room; he hopped in on one foot and then the other, falling this way and that as he tried to balance. Then he ran around madly while the other children took their seats. The teaching assistant directed him to his chair but he did not sit on it; instead he used it to vault across the table.

'Please sit down, Benjamin,' said the teacher in a tone that suggested she said this a hundred times a day.

Benjamin ran around the classroom again and finally sat down. But he could not sit still. The other children listened while he fidgeted, flicked his pencil across the room, retrieved it, flicked it further.

The teacher turned to him. 'I've asked you, Benjamin, not to do that. Now let's see how you get on with the maths problem. Remember, everyone, you can't touch any of the shapes which are red . . .'

Benjamin showed a flicker of interest in the shapes. For a moment they became the focus of his considerable energy. There was the low hum of voices collaborating all around the room. Except at Benjamin's table, where there was silence. He had taken all the shapes and was trying by himself, with a speed that invalidated the attempt, to fit them together. Of course, he was touching the red ones, flipping them around the table. I felt sorry for the other children in his group, but they waited patiently, as though they knew he would soon lose interest. And he did. He could sit no longer. He leapt to his feet and began doing star jumps.

I stayed until lunchtime. The last thing I saw was Benjamin, unable to focus on his meal for long enough to eat it, leaping up to do star jumps between mouthfuls.

'What do you think?' asked his teacher.

'I'm new to the clinic. I'm usually an adult psychiatrist. I have to say I've never seen anything like it and I don't know how you cope.'

She smiled. 'It's a real challenge. Today the other children were quite well-behaved, maybe because you were observing us. But it's not always that way. I've seen them recoil from Benjamin and his behaviour. There's name-calling and some very unkind comments. And now a few boys are trying to fight him, physically. I have to check for bullying all the time. I used to think Benjamin was just naughty but after a while I could see it was something much more than that.'

'It isn't easy for anyone being in Benjamin's class,' I said. 'A few children have been taken out by their parents.' She looked tired. 'I really hope you can help him.'

'Well?' asked the professor as soon as I was back in the clinic.

'Okay, I take back what I said about ADHD being no more than a fashionable diagnosis. It exists. I saw it today.'

'How do they cope with him in class?'

'They're brilliant. But, to be frank, there's no coping with him.'

He looked at me intently. 'I can change Benjamin. I can change what life is like for everyone around him. I can change his relationships, his academic achievement, I can make him happier. But it does mean prescribing amphetamine salts. Still think I shouldn't?'

I backed down, of course. Although I wondered if anyone or anything could help a kid like Benjamin. He came to the clinic, we formally diagnosed him with ADHD and he immediately started stimulant medication.

I spent the next six months at the clinic and found working with children fascinating and challenging. It did not occur to me, however, that one day I would specialize in child psychiatry. At that stage, ADHD was just a part of a whole new world and I wanted to explore every continent.

Towards the end of my placement, I went back to Benjamin's school. It was the summer term now. The children had taken off their sweatshirts and their clothes lay in jumbled piles across the playground: kids dodged them as they ran around in shirt sleeves. It was even harder to get to the entrance this time. It seemed to me that either the children had all grown or the playground was smaller.

The same receptionist let me in. 'You came before, you're on the professor's team. Well, from everyone here, I say a big thank you.'

The teacher said: 'I don't know what you've given him. At first I thought you must have sedated him.'

'Oh no,' I assured her.

'Well, whatever it is, you've changed my life! I'm not sure I could have coped with him for much longer.'

And when the children filed in, Benjamin was among them but the teacher had to remind me which child he was. He sat down with the others, opened his book, studied it, put his hand up to answer questions. And then, most remarkable of all, he sat with his pencil in his hand, concentrating hard on his workbook. He was entirely unrecognizable.

'How's he doing academically?' I asked.

'Oh, very well. I always knew he was extremely bright, but getting him to concentrate long enough to learn anything was almost impossible. And there's one other important change. I don't think Benjamin enjoyed being the way he was. He was always on the edge of being bullied because there was clearly something wrong with him and you know what kids are like when they work out someone's different.'

Yup. I knew.

'He had no friends before, really. And now he's got lots. Overall, he's so much happier.'

Working in that clinic with the professor was an extraordinary experience for me because I felt as though I was making children better and improving the quality of their lives exponentially. Yes, it was true that elsewhere too many kids were told for the wrong reasons that they had ADHD and, yes, too many of them were taking stimulant medication. But I knew now that there was a hard core of children who suffered from a genuinely unmanageable condition and the right medication could change their trajectory.

So, from being passionately against them, I now believed passionately in giving some children medical stimulants. It was to be some years before my views changed again.

6

I was thirty-seven, both practising psychiatry and lecturing in it, when I took my final exams for admittance to the Royal College of Psychiatrists. And it was around this time that I first encountered forensic patients. These are patients who have already, or might, commit a crime.

I was working on a high-intensity ward. Todd was transferred to us from prison. His behaviour there had become so erratic that the prison psychologist had been concerned. Was he psychotic? He had been seen by the prison psychiatrist, who thought he was. Todd was then detained under the Mental Health Act and had now arrived in our hospital for a fuller assessment.

He was on remand for rape. He had moved into that grey area where the criminal justice system and the health service overlap.

Except, I thought he was pretending to be psychotic.

'Yep, doc, I'm certainly seeing things. Aaaargh! There's one now!'

'One what, Todd?'

'One of the big, hairy things that keeps appearing . . . can't you see him too? You must be able to see his teeth.'

'No. Where is he?'

'Right over there. Aaaargh! On the ceiling.'

I certainly did not bother to turn around and check the ceiling. Instead, I studied Todd closely. Was that the flicker of a half-smile? Until now, not many of my patients had been feigning mental illness. Most of them went to great lengths to hide it. I said nothing. And wondered how I should deal with this.

Very soon after Todd was admitted, I attended a meeting for psychiatrists (these are frequent) and met a doctor called John Brontë. He specialized in cases like Todd's: he was a forensic psychiatrist. In fact, he had qualified as a forensic psychiatrist for children as well as adults, so he encountered offenders of all ages.

His work was so different from my general psychiatry that it seemed we were unlikely to meet again, anyway professionally. But we greatly liked each other. He was older than me. His hair was pure white, although he had a youthful vigour. He spoke about his work with passion. I wondered if he was anyone's father and thought how lucky they were. I'd spent much of my childhood wishing Dr Who was my father. I'd given that up now, although I certainly hadn't given up *Dr Who*.

John liked whisky and we found ourselves in a pub together after the meeting.

He took a sip of whisky and sighed with satisfaction. 'So, you're asking why this patient would pretend to be mentally ill when you really don't think he is? Well, that's a problem I encounter on a regular basis. As does any forensic psychiatrist.'

'You mean, people who've committed a crime try to say they're ill so it wasn't their fault?'

It's hard to believe now that I was so naïve. John laughed and told me that offenders can dramatically reduce their time in jail, especially if their crime is homicide, by proving the crime is linked to a psychiatric condition.

'And,' he added, 'don't forget that, once an offender is convicted, being ill can secure them a stay on a hospital ward, which some may find a lot more pleasant than prison. So that's a good reason to pretend to be ill. But before their trial and sentence, well, that's of course when I face the greatest risk of deception.'

'Todd isn't actually convicted of this crime, although I gather he's spent time in prison for rape before. He's on remand, waiting for his trial.'

'And I understand he's convinced a prison psychiatrist to diagnose him?'

I nodded.

'Well then, he might be looking for some sentencing leniency. Hoping that the court will think that, if he's psychotic now, then he must have been psychotic if and when he committed the crime.'

I thought forensic work must be like cat and mouse, trying to assess people who were setting out to deceive you. I imagined prisoners studying psychology books in their cells to make their performances more authentic.

'That's where training and experience come in. Every patient is a challenge: some have committed terrible crimes and it's my job to make sense of that within a mental health context. There's so much confusion and deception with these complex cases: I have to bring some clarity to the court.'

What must it be like to deal daily with people who had killed, raped and maimed other people? To sit talking with aggressive, threatening men of the kind I would cross the street to avoid? What would you find inside their heads?

John said: 'I certainly swim in murky waters, but I love it. Truly love it. Yes, a lot of the patients have committed appalling crimes. And I'm locked in a cell-like room interviewing them closely for many hours. But I'm doing that in order to see the world through their eyes. Only then can I begin to understand.'

I found myself both scared and fascinated by the idea. Repelled and drawn to it.

John said: 'Remember, only a small proportion of patients is trying to fool me. Many are really very ill. In the criminal justice system you will find a wide and truly extraordinary range of psychiatric and neurodiverse conditions. Many of these cannot be treated or even alleviated and that's something a forensic psychiatrist has to come to terms with.'

'I'm already coming to terms with it in general psychiatry.'

John took a sip of whisky and paused again to enjoy it. Then he said: 'My job is quite different from yours. I don't actually treat patients, not unless I especially want to. Mostly I assess them. I assess whether they are fit to plead guilty or not guilty. I assess whether they are mentally ill now. I assess whether they were mentally ill at the time of the crime. I write detailed reports on this for the court. Sometimes I recommend courses which may help them: educational or rehabilitation courses. Sometimes I recommend treatment. But as a forensic psychiatrist, I seldom actually treat patients myself. I hope this doesn't sound immodest, but I'm past that. I can do more good in this world by diagnosing and understanding what might help patients – and then handing them to others for treatment.'

'So you spend a lot of your time writing about your cases?'

'In considerable detail.'

Forensic psychiatry was certainly not for me. I still wanted to make as many people better as possible, not sit around writing long, tedious reports all day.

John laughed.

'Patients are never, ever tedious. I see a lot of children and how can that be dull? Remember, I'm assessing, not treating, and my reports are analytical, unlike the discharge notes you write. Duncan, I know you're finishing general psychiatry soon: if you're looking to specialize, you should consider the forensic world.'

I shook my head. No way. It was too scary to think of working closely with such dangerous individuals, talking to them about the hideous, violent, cruel things they had done. Locked in a room with men who were adult, more threatening versions of the school bullies I remembered so well. Men who were like my father. And as for being a child forensic psychiatrist like John, well, just imagine all those unreasoning, knife-wielding, monosyllabic teenagers. Nope. Not for me.

I returned to the ward and observed Todd and decided that, although he was aggressive to staff and other patients, there were no evident symptoms of psychosis. He was violent, not psychotic. Medication was not required. I wrote his discharge report. He went back to prison. But this was an interesting, unusual case for me and I found myself giving John Brontë's words a lot of thought.

A few months later, the police appeared. The two officers, one female, one male, arrived on the ward looking large in their uniforms. They took off their hats, and their hats looked large too. The patients knew they were here in the office and I was aware of a flutter of consternation out there followed by an unusual silence.

The female officer was friendly and smiling. Did I remember a patient called Angus Radinksi?

I had to think hard. This was a very busy ward and, once a patient had been discharged, they were immediately replaced by another. I turned the screen so the police officers could not see it and took a quick look at his notes. Ah yes. A big, brooding man who had been admitted through A&E after an attempted suicide. There had been a major relationship break-up and he had tried to hang himself, unsuccessfully (one thing I had learned by now was that death by hanging is not easily achieved). His depression was certainly acute and he had been very silent. We had treated him and released him to community health services after a week. I hoped the police weren't here to say he had killed himself.

I didn't tell the officers any of this, of course: I wasn't sure how much confidential information I could reveal, even to the police.

The male officer smiled less than his colleague. He said seriously: 'We understand that he was discharged from this ward about a month ago?'

I nodded. Yes, I could say that much.

'Unfortunately, he's nearly killed a man. Went into a shop to buy a bottle of beer, didn't have quite enough money on him. The shopkeeper wouldn't let him have the beer for a few pence less than the price. He smashed the beer, went out, and, before the shopkeeper could clear up, came back with a claw hammer.'

I winced. 'Did he . . . ?'

'Yes,' said the woman officer. We all looked thoroughly miserable now. 'Went for the shopkeeper's face. Life-changing injuries. 'Nuff said.'

'We've got him locked up,' added her colleague, 'but we know he's got mental health difficulties and we'll need any information you can give us.'

I said: 'I can't give you anything specific right now. In fact, I'm honestly not sure exactly what I can say.' I thought of the shopkeeper who would not sell his beer for a few pennies under its price. He had lost so much more than pennies. 'But,' I added, 'I'll try to have a summary report ready for you very quickly.'

My supervisor suggested that I contact the forensic department, as they had originally assessed this patient over a year ago. I phoned them at once.

'I'm the one you want to talk to, come right down!' said a cheerful senior registrar. 'Bring us both a coffee, and don't forget your notebook.'

I descended to the basement where my forensic colleagues worked. Their offices were so low in the hospital that the only light source was far above eye level, reinforcing the impression that I had plunged to murky depths.

'Does your job ever depress you?' I asked the registrar. He looked ordinary enough, nothing like as morose as you would expect of someone dealing all day with people who didn't think twice before they reached for the claw hammer.

He grinned at me the way John Brontë had.

'You get used to it. They're patients to me, not murderers. Basically, I think this is the most interesting department in the hospital . . . Now, you're enquiring about Angus Radinski, is that correct?'

He started to talk to me about Radinski. Whereas I was pushed to remember any details about the man, the registrar seemed to have total recall. I took notes.

'Well, at first his criminal history followed a familiar pattern: started as a teenager with a bit of street robbery, progressed to robbing houses, then to aggravated burglaries, then to taking vehicles without consent, then, I think, to knife-carrying. Nothing unusual about that, except that he had been treated during this period for severe depression. In his mid-twenties there was a lull when he got a job and seemed to settle down. That lasted into his thirties if I remember rightly, until he was about thirty-three a year or so ago. Then we became involved.'

I scribbled frantically, trying to keep up.

'His neighbours called the police because they heard screaming and banging and yelling coming from the Radinski flat . . . and, sure enough, his partner was found badly bleeding and beaten up with the tell-tale marks of a ligature around her neck. He was arrested and we were called in to assess him.'

'Called in where?' I asked. I was enthralled.

'To prison.'

'Are you called in every time someone's arrested for domestic abuse?'

'Good God, no. But Angus had a history of mental health problems; he'd actually been seen by the community team when he was committing burglaries, back when he was suffering from depression. The police saw this on his record and thought they needed him assessed now.'

'But . . . what were you assessing him for?'

'Evidence of mental disorder. Was he fit for a police interview? Fit to plead guilty or not guilty? Fit to stand trial? After an attack on his partner like that – and I believe he was close to killing her – I'd have to start by looking for psychosis, of course.'

'You went into a cell and talked to him about strangling his wife?'

'Talked to him about a lot of things. This was an assessment.'

'Just you and him?'

'Yep, without so much as a panic button. It can be quite frightening.'

I felt that mixture of fascination and horror I had experienced when I was talking to John Brontë. And I remembered feeling it before. On my arrival at medical school, when we had started to cut up dead bodies. At first, I had wanted to run out of the lab, but eventually I had become so absorbed that nothing could have dragged me away.

'And so . . .' I asked breathlessly. 'Was Angus Radinksi psychotic?'

'In my opinion he was not psychotic, not depressed, not mentally ill at all.'

'And if he had been?'

'I would have had him transferred to hospital and instigated a much fuller assessment. But there was nothing wrong with him. So he had to stay out of hospital and in the criminal justice system and I could give the police the go-ahead to get on with their job.'

'What happened to him? I suppose he was jailed?'

'Nope. Because the partner dropped charges.'

'He'd tried to throttle her and she dropped charges?'

'It's very common in domestic abuse cases. There are so many different pressures on the victim. So many fears, so many emotions.'

'What happened to him?'

'Well, sometimes the police manage to continue with a prosecution even when charges have been dropped by the victim. But not this time. Because his partner now claimed someone in the street had tried to strangle her and Angus had simply been helping her. That was almost certainly not true. But what could the police do about it? Nothing.'

'So he nearly killed a woman but he was released?'

'Yep. He's dangerous. I would say that the recent claw hammer incident is a likely part of his trajectory. But look, we did remain open to him for six months, and support services were offered to the partner. No one was engaging with us chez Radinski, though. So, based on information you've given me, it looks as though it took eight months for the partner to ditch him and six months after that for him to attempt suicide and gain admittance to your ward.'

I had hardly noticed this patient. Another depression, another suicide. Now I realized there was so much more to be known about him. If only there was time.

'Was his childhood difficult?'

'Oh yes, mother abandoned him when he was about three. Literally. He and his little sister were found in a flat half starving and taken into care. The mother occasionally reappeared to disrupt his life, insisting that she wanted her son to live with her, but she was neglectful – reading between the lines, I think she may have had an addiction problem – anyway, his stays with Mum always ended disastrously and he'd go back into care.'

'So . . . you could understand where this criminal trajectory came from?'

His eyes strayed to the light that was tipping in from one wall high above us.

'Understand, yes. The question is, how far do we treat a difficult childhood as an excuse for crime? I can understand that, after his mother abandoning him, his partner leaving might have triggered his suicide attempt. But do we really think that makes it okay to get out the claw hammer?'

'Did he receive any help?'

'You mean, psychotherapy? I don't know. I doubt it.'

'So . . . when did you personally last see him?'

'Oh . . . between a year and eighteen months ago.'

I nodded. 'I guess you looked all this up after I rang you. Although I don't know how you had time to read the file.' It had only taken me five minutes to buy coffees and find the forensic psychiatry unit.

'No, no, I haven't looked anything up,' he assured me. 'I probably should do that now. I've just been telling you everything I remember.'

I was stunned.

'But . . . you saw him more than a year ago!'

'Seems like yesterday.'

'How can you possibly remember everything? Are you one of those people who wins memory competitions?'

He laughed.

'I could supply you with a lot of detail on any patient, going back years. So could all my colleagues in this department.'

'Do they give you a memory test before they let you into forensics?'

He laughed again.

'That's the difference between you and me. You have so many patients you can't remember any of them. For me, it's about the depth.'

I tried to remember a patient. Any patient. Ah, Petra, the woman with bipolar affective disorder who had gone shopping one day and come home with a digger. She was an early case and there had been no psychologist available so I had talked to her for longer than most and begun to understand her relatively well. That was how I had known that releasing her would have disastrous consequences for her, whatever the tribunal said. Since then, though, I had been much more superficial and detached in my dealings with patients. Because there was no expectation, and certainly no time, to be anything else.

The registrar said: 'Forensic psychiatrists work in considerable depth. I interview for hours, often more than once, and write very, very detailed reports for the court. So detailed that I remember everything I say.'

I was incredulous. And then jealous. I wanted the registrar's job. I imagined spending hours with a patient, going into great detail. Then sitting in my home office at night, watched over, from the shelf on the wall, by the silent figures of Dr Who and my other old friend, Tintin, while I wrote considered reports.

For the police, I put together just a couple of paragraphs on Angus Radinski. I doubt it had much significance for them, but for me this case was important. It was my first real encounter with forensic psychiatry and I had been both horrified and seduced by it.

'The registrar remembered everything!' I told John Brontë. 'He knew all about the patient although he hadn't opened the file for a year. And he'd given the case so much thought.'

John said: 'Yes. That's the way it is in forensic psychiatry.'

He had invited me to his home. Glancing into the other old houses in the same street, I had seen that many lacked internal walls: they were open plan, expanded at the back by glassy, boxy structures. In John's house, no walls had been knocked down. It had an almost labyrinthine collection of small rooms and there was not a glass box but a back door to the garden. Now we were sitting under a shady tree on the lawn.

'I'm getting really frustrated at work,' I said. 'I know I have to specialize soon, and I'm sure I don't want to stay in general psychiatry. The patients are in and out, in and out; I feel as if I'm living in a revolving door. In community services there's a burgeoning case list. And I'm always dashing to A&E to meet someone else I don't really have time to talk to . . . I'm constantly fighting fires and never really getting to know a single patient.'

He nodded receptively, a professional sort of nod.

'So, when I talked to the registrar in the forensic department and he had total recall of just one patient, I really began to wonder . . .'

I paused. I did not know what I was about to say.

'I really began to wonder if forensic psychiatry might be for me.'

I stared at John in surprise, as if the words had not been mine but his.

John looked at me wisely. 'Yes. I thought so.'

'Did you?'

'Yes, from the moment I met you.'

'Really?'

'Yes. I'd be pleased to mentor you through this process.'

Suddenly I was delighted. The ugliness and brutality of crime which had horrified me at first had turned into a mystery to be solved, a human mind to be understood, a puzzle to be unlocked. And maybe, just maybe, it might be possible to help people turn their lives around and move away from crime. Yes, even after my failure to rid the world of polio, I still harboured that kind of fantasy. Plus, John would be there to help me.

'But . . . where do I start?'

'Hmmm. There's a process . . . you've just passed your exams for the Royal College of Psychiatrists so you can make the relevant applications to specialize. But perhaps you should dip your toe in the water first. With a placement at the Personality Disorder Unit.'

I looked around at John's flowering shrubs. The lawn was closely mown and the edges were neat but the shrubs tumbled in all directions: some could hardly bear the weight of their flowers.

'Why there?'

'It's highly forensic. Should give you a very good idea of what you're getting yourself into.'

7

My first few months on the Personality Disorder Unit were quiet because none of the patients spoke to me. Some of them had committed extremely violent crimes. Others were smooth-talking paedophiles. Most were simply dangerous.

They were all being held against their will. Many had served sentences but now they were here on restrictive court orders for public safety. So they were effectively prisoners, but for us they were patients. And this was a therapeutic ward. Meaning that the patients were seldom confined to cells but were free to interact with each other and staff in a manner which was supposed, 24/7, to be a therapeutic environment: an environment less like prison and more like the world out there that they might soon be joining.

I wasn't sure it really worked that way, though. It was not easy for staff to interact all the time with so many dangerous, violent, unpredictable men. So they tended to gravitate to the nurses' station rather than talking with patients.

I, personally, did not always feel safe as the patients sidled around me suspiciously, never meeting my eye, pretending to ignore me but watching me with curiosity whenever my back was turned. It was part of my job to carry out mental and physical health assessments and write regular reports and reviews for the Ministry of Justice. This is essential when people are held against their will. In addition, I was doctor for the ward's various ailments, however minor – the ingrowing toenails and the bruised elbows.

After a few months of deep suspicion, patients began to bring me their minor medical problems and I gradually got to know them. I was keen. Soon I was training to participate in some of the many rehabilitation programmes. I was especially interested in the violence reduction programme which was gaining favour at the time and soon I started to work with individual patients.

Together we would build a framework of understanding. We might discuss a news story initially. Nothing involving crime, though, more likely a story about, for instance, someone protesting against a new government policy. Why wasn't the policy working for them? Why had it been implemented? How did the people affected by the policy actually feel?

Next we might move on to discussing small decisions they themselves made in the course of a day. How did they talk to other patients? Should they retaliate if someone threatened or annoyed them? And then: how much of that decision-making was based on what they thought the other person was experiencing? What tiny ripples and repercussions might result from their action? And what further decision-making situations might now arise?

Eventually, we would reach the right point to discuss how the victims of their crimes might have felt. It was useless to start with that. You had to creep slowly towards it.

I got to know and even like some of the patients. Adam

had borderline personality disorder, now known in the UK as emotionally unstable personality disorder. His offences were extremely violent. He had been subjected to shocking neglect, abuse and violence in his childhood and, put simply, now he externalized that by hurting others – and also internalized it by hurting himself. He could be smart, funny and good company. If you could ignore the open wounds which he would never allow to heal. His scabs were always picked and reopened and enlarged, and I tried not to look at them when I talked to the interesting and thoughtful Adam.

One day I received an emergency call. There was a riot on the ward. Police and tactical support were there but things were out of control.

I was lecturing elsewhere at the time. I got around London on a motorbike in those days and now I abandoned my students, jumped on the bike and whizzed off.

As I reached the gates, I was flagged down by a police officer. I assumed that, as his colleagues were waiting for me on the other side of the gates, he was directing me. But no.

'Do you realize just what speed you were going, sir?'

I tried to explain that this was an emergency, but ward riots were of little interest to him. He insisted on delivering a lecture and handing me a ticket. A procedure which he stretched to about twenty minutes – deliberately, it seemed to me. He ignored my pleas to contact his colleagues.

When I finally rode through the gates, there were fire engines and police officers everywhere and the whole site was in lockdown. Lights flashed, buzzers buzzed, officers stared at me.

They said: 'This is an emergency, you said you were nearby, what took you so long?'

No point explaining. Later, I appealed my fine, but was still forced to pay it.

'What's happening?' I asked everyone, breathlessly.

'It's all under control now. Except for one of them.'

'What's his name?'

'Adam.'

An officer told me what had happened. The nursing stations were small rooms within rooms and the men had waited until all the nurses were huddled together inside, as they so often were. Then the patients had crawled under the nursing station windows so they wouldn't be spotted and rapidly shut the door. Before any staff could realize what was happening and escape, they had superglued the lock. Finally, they had kicked the surrounding doors to jam the locks before setting fire to the nursing station. With five nurses inside.

When I entered the ward it was bedlam, with upturned chairs, paperwork strewn across the floor, burn marks on the walls and a nursing station which looked as if it had half melted. The nurses had been badly frightened, and perhaps angered, but, thank heavens, not physically hurt. Security was too efficient for that. The most unpalatable fact by far was that Adam had tried to burn five people alive. Adam, with whom I had been discussing only yesterday how to make decisions which considered the feelings of others.

He was regarded as one of two ringleaders and had been detained in a seclusion room by the police. So had the other leader. And when that man was told to take off his clothes, he produced a lighter from an orifice and calmly set fire to the room. Adam had also been hiding something which he produced when he was told to take off his clothes. A razor blade. Yesterday we had also been talking intensely about not harming himself as well as others and all the time a razor blade had been hidden deep inside one of his wounds.

He announced to the police that he was going to eat the razor blade. And did. They watched, horrified, as he chewed and then swallowed it, blood issuing from his mouth.

Wondering when the doctor was going to arrive, they told him they were taking him straight to A&E. He refused. No. He would not go to A&E, he was staying right here. He had already been Sectioned into this ward and he now calmly pointed out that the Section was applicable to his mental and not physical health and no one had the right to make him go anywhere.

'Get him to say he'll go to the fucking hospital!' a police officer instructed me as I entered.

Adam stood there, naked and silent.

'What was it all about, Adam?' My voice was gentle. He did not look at me.

He said little but I gathered that the patients had quietly declared war on the staff when a secret hooch-making operation had been discovered and stopped. However, this was no time for us to unpick the riot. I wanted him to go to A&E.

I asked him nicely, but he shook his head. I tried every tactic I knew short of pleading. He would not budge. My job was then to decide whether he had the mental capacity to make the decision to stay here. If he did not, then the police would have to take him forcibly.

I asked to take a look at his mouth and he agreed. I discovered that only the lip was slightly cut. I didn't know how someone could chew on a razor blade and still have a tongue, but there were no visible wounds inside the mouth itself. I asked how he was feeling and he said he was fine. No pain in his throat or stomach.

I decided that he had mental capacity to make this decision. He stayed in segregation and was watched carefully and we all learned that, incredibly, you could chew and swallow a razor blade without causing any apparent harm.

The ward gradually returned to its usual calm, the strained sort of calm when everyone is always ready for a serious incident. Now that I had been there a while and patients were more relaxed around me, my naïve, bouncing enthusiasm was beginning to wane. A lot of them wanted to talk to me these days, talk about themselves and about their crimes in considerable detail.

At first I was pleased. But I was starting to wonder if this was part of a more insidious process. Was it possible that some patients derived pleasure from reliving their crimes and registering any distaste or shock I might show, no matter how hard I tried to hide it? And was I in some way allowing myself to be infiltrated by their mixture of cruelty and madness and their need to deposit it somewhere? I was still inexperienced and some patients surely knew that I had not yet learned defensive mechanisms.

This was true of no one more than Joseph. He had started by bringing a physical ailment to me – oddly, it was his thumb – and, when we stopped talking about his thumb, we started talking about Joseph.

He was a serial paedophile. He had been released from prison by the Parole Board and immediately reoffended. Now he had completed his sentence but was stuck in the system. Something was preventing his progression towards release and that was Joseph's inability to feel any empathy for his victims.

He was charming, clever and entertaining and I was pleased to do some individual work with him. He became my project.

I knew I couldn't 'cure' him; he would always be attracted to children. But I hoped that our sessions might prompt some kind of regret and understanding of his crime, even a determination not to act on his needs. This might lead to the ultimate goal: safe release.

'Actually, Doc . . .' Joseph was a handsome, middle-aged man. This was our eighth session and now he leaned forward and a lock of grey hair fell across his face. He looked shy and boyish for a moment. 'I've drafted Charlotte a letter.'

Charlotte was one of his victims. She had been nine when Joseph had charmed her parents. This had given him open access to their daughter, whom he had first groomed and then raped. It hadn't felt like rape to Joseph. He had told himself it was a loving, giving thing to do and that Charlotte had enjoyed it. Now Charlotte was in her twenties. Joseph had certainly caused her irreparable harm. And he wanted to write to her.

'I've written that I hope she's okay, how bad I feel about it all and how sorry I am. Want to read it?'

'No, Joseph,' I said gently.

'Why not?'

This was not victim empathy. This was, in a different way, another attempt to violate her. Whatever equilibrium she had eventually achieved in her life, Joseph's letter could destroy it. And I thought that, deep down, he must know that.

'Let's think how Charlotte might feel on receiving a letter from you. Writing it might make you feel better. But what about her?'

He paused and his face creased along his wrinkle lines, as if a diner was refolding a napkin after a meal.

'You mean . . . I shouldn't send it? You think she'd mind?'

'I'm absolutely sure you shouldn't send it.'

Joseph gave me a look of such injury and misery, as if everything was my fault, that I really felt terrible. I even considered for a moment whether there were circumstances in which I could ease his pain by allowing him to send the letter. A part of me knew that this was the sort of manipulation one might expect of someone with his mental condition and a part of me was actually manipulated. Thank heavens I was going to see John Brontë that very evening.

8

I always looked forward to sitting down and talking with the man who had slowly become my friend, teacher and mentor. We had seen each other often, heard each other's stories and knew each other well by now.

My head was throbbing as I wove my way on my motorbike through the London traffic. I could feel the winter wind buffeting me. When I stopped at traffic lights, I watched people's necks disappearing into their coats as they crossed the road, faces down. I watched them without seeing them. I knew that Joseph was still inside my head, and the psychiatrist's head is not a good place for a patient to hang around.

'Hmmm,' said my mentor, studying me as I took off my helmet. 'I think you need Dr Brontë's prescription.'

He poured us both a whisky and we sank into armchairs in front of the fire in his study. The curtains were drawn, the room was warm. I held up my glass and looked at the fire through the whisky. I had never liked to tell John this, but I preferred looking at whisky to drinking it. The colour was so beautiful. I had seen nothing beautiful all day in the Personality Disorder Unit. It was a battered, tired, ugly place, full of angry people who were quite capable of spitting at you or throwing faeces in your face, and sometimes did.

'Head still banging away?' John asked sympathetically.

I was so used to the strange throbbing in my head – it

had started some years ago – that I had hardly noticed it today.

'It never really stops banging these days. It's just worse sometimes than others. I'm not even sure if it's my ear or my head.'

He nodded and waited and I told him about Joseph.

'What did you hope to achieve by doing this individual work with him?' he asked.

'I thought he might be able to understand how much harm he's caused his victims.'

I wondered how Charlotte had coped as she had grown in years and understanding, as she had developed sexually. How had she made sense of her relationship with Joseph? How had she managed her adult sexual relationships? She had been skilfully groomed by Joseph, and groomed children usually believe that what happened with their abuser was entirely their fault. Charlotte was certainly a rape victim, but it might have taken many years for her to realize that – if she ever did.

'Deep down, Joseph still believes that a nine-year-old seduced him,' I said. 'That he had a truly loving relationship with her because that's what she wanted. And he probably persuaded Charlotte to believe it too.'

'Let's see, you've had . . . how many sessions with him now?'

'Eight.'

'Good gracious. Isn't it time you produced a report?'

'I'll do it soon. And it will say he's not able to experience true, deep-down empathy for others or genuine regret for the pain he's caused. I'll have to say that he might abuse again if he's released. And then he'll read it and be bitterly disappointed and then I'll have to discuss it with him and then we'll be on suicide watch. Actually, I can hardly face discussing it with him.'

'But you must discuss it, Duncan. You must explain to him that unless he can understand the harm he did to those children, then he's at risk of abusing again on release.'

I thought how Joseph's hair would hang sadly across his brow in a single curl and his face would crease and he might even cry.

'He's going to feel so hurt. As if I've betrayed him.'

'Joseph's good at making everyone else think things are their fault. Now, if you're worrying that doing the right thing will hurt him then I'm afraid you're not really observing strict enough boundaries.'

It was true. I resolved then and there to end the sessions, write my report, discuss it with Joseph. And move on.

'I really thought I could help him,' I said sadly.

'Perhaps you have. It may show over time.'

I sighed.

John was watching me closely. 'Why does this man get under your skin? It is, of course, the particular skill of anyone in the Personality Disorder Unit to do that. But you know you could and should have stopped his sessions by now.'

'He's highly intelligent, humorous, entertaining . . .' I rearranged myself in my chair and swilled my whisky around in the glass. 'I hate to say it, but he can be very good company. And the bespoke work we're doing is a significant part of his violence reduction programme.'

'Duncan. Please. I asked why he gets under your skin.'

I paused.

'I find myself liking him. Until he starts to give me a graphic account of how he raped children.'

'So here's a man you rather like who does terrible things.'

'The whole ward is that way. A lot of the patients are really likeable and clever. But they're also highly volatile, hard to predict, very violent and some are downright scary.'

He said: 'Just like your dad.'

Then he sipped his whisky and looked at the fire.

I stared back at the fire as if John's face was there. No, as if my dad's face was there. His mouth a big, black O, his moustache almost standing on end with fury. The fire hissed and I heard his terrible scream. The one that meant he was having a seizure and would soon be beating up anyone in his path. I was not his small son; I was nothing more than a skittle. I felt his fist meet my face and my body collapse on to the sofa, wanting to keep my eyes shut so that I would not see him hurling my mother across the room, her legs flopping like a rag doll's. There was the terrible crash of her callipers. I opened my eyes. She lay silently on the floor, elbows out, neck askew, her metal legs flung at unnatural, acute angles.

'Duncan . . .' a kind voice, speaking from a great distance, decades away. 'Have you ever talked to anyone about your father? Your parents?'

I shook my head.

'Perhaps you should?' John said kindly. 'Especially now that you're working with such violent patients.'

I blinked at him. I couldn't actually see the connection between a childhood with my violent father and a working life with my patients. I tried to sound reasonable. 'John, really, what does my job have to do with my dad?'

Well, that was a stupid question and as soon as I heard it I knew as much. As if we don't all internalize our parents and carry them around inside us throughout our lives.

John smiled at the fire.

'So you made a choice to become a forensic psychiatrist. You're starting your first placement soon and the PD Unit is your kindergarten. But even here you're surrounded by extremely dangerous men and, from now on, you will be. And yet you haven't asked yourself why you've chosen a branch of medicine that brings you into contact with these people?'

I swallowed. No, I had not asked myself that. I had simply thought that travelling through the minds of offenders was the most interesting job I could ever do and that forensic psychiatry might be a place where I could really help people – not just the patient, but wider society.

'In a professional capacity,' he continued calmly, 'you will understand scary, abusive men; perhaps you will answer the question: why? And maybe even help them change.'

My mouth was dry. I took a huge gulp of whisky. It burned my throat as if I had swallowed not the whisky but the fire.

He said: 'You want to understand violence. And perhaps control it. Which, of course, you longed to do as a child.'

My parents split up and came together and split up again through my childhood, like the tributaries of some old river. I was powerless to influence the river's course. The night that ended it all came when I was about five. Dad returned late from the pub. My mother prepared tea in angry silence. I knew the food would taste of anger.

When he arrived, Dad seemed not to notice her fury. His face was bright red and he chatted all through the meal, asking me a question and, a few minutes later, asking me again. I glanced at Mum and answered each time.

He tried talking to Mum. She would not look at him and she would not reply. I felt more and more tense. I knew that something awful would follow.

Mum had made apple crumble. It was sweet and delicious, crunchy on top with the softness of the apple beneath. I tried to think only of crumble but the room was changing. As if a new person, a big, angry person who we couldn't see, had walked in and sat down at the table.

'You didn't make a good job of peeling the apples,' said Dad, leaning back in his chair. 'There are some nasty hard bits of skin in here.'

My mother stood up.

She moved towards him. Donk, swish, click.

She leaned on one crutch.

She raised the other one above his head.

'Fuck you!' she screamed.

The crutch crashed down hard on Dad. The crutches were not heavy, not like callipers. I thought: if Mum had hit Dad with her callipers then he would probably be dead. And for a moment, a terrible moment, I wished he was.

I doubted that the crutch had hurt him very much. But that was not the point. The point was that she had hit him.

I waited in horror for what would happen next.

Dad's red face grew bigger. Bigger than a balloon and then bigger than a sunset. When he stood up, his whole body swelled until he filled the room, his head pressing against the ceiling, his arms against the walls. And Mum looked very, very small.

They were both shouting. They were so loud that I could not hear them. Then Dad picked up Mum. Her skirt fluttered and her legs, her callipers, her boots, all hung from just one of his arms, like washing. He was going to hang out the washing and the washing was Mum.

He threw her as hard as he could at the plate glass of the kitchen door. There was a hideous sound. The door smashing, Mum smashing, the whole world smashing into small pieces as she crashed through it and lay still on the other side.

Dad stumbled around, breaking anything he could. Bowls of apple crumble landed on the walls, plates disintegrated into the sink. He found a knife, the one Mum had used to cut the vegetables, and threw it at her. It missed and bounced on the hall carpet.

I was so frightened that I could not think at all. My heartbeat deafened me. Dad stormed into the lounge and I heard such a big crash that I knew this must be the TV. I grabbed my chance and ran to the open door. My feet crunched on glass. Mum was lying in a pool of glass and blood. I knelt at her side and felt the warm blood seeping through the knees of my trousers.

'Fucking bastard,' moaned Mum.

She was alive!

'Get out,' she whispered to me. 'Now. I mean it, now.'

I saw, lying by her side, the knife Dad had thrown. He could still kill her with it. I grabbed it and slipped out of the front door.

The street was quiet. No traffic, just the weird orange of streetlamps making everything a different colour from the daytime. I looked down at my trousers. They were damp with Mum's blood but under the lights the blood was purple. My knees felt cold in the night air. I sensed movement in neighbours' windows, swift and short.

I walked up the hill. My head was empty. I was shaking so much that I got down on to my wet knees and felt the hardness of the tarmac. It was impossible to stop shaking just by trying. My teeth chattered, my whole body rattled, inside and out, like a toy train going off the track.

In the distance, then closer, then right by me, was a loud whine. I could feel the car's blue light fall across my face. Footsteps. Voices. Someone picked up the knife, which was lying in the road beside me. Light spilled suddenly out of our house, as if it had been leaning against the door when someone opened it.

'Let's get you off the road, love, and somewhere we can keep you nice and warm.' The policewoman's face was shielded by her hat..

She talked to me softly. I could make no sense of her words, but I could feel her kindness. When we were sitting in the back of a police car together, I saw her in the street light. She had big, black eyes.

She gave me hot chocolate from a flask. I stared at it and then tasted it and when I'd tasted it then I wanted to drink it. She winked at me and produced a small plastic bag. Marshmallows. She gave me one and its softness exploded into sweetness in my mouth.

She smiled and offered me another. I had stopped shaking now. I didn't want to think and I didn't want to talk.

'Ambulance is taking her in, the lad's going to her father's,' said a policeman, who had been talking on a radio and was now getting into the car.

We set off and the policewoman said kindly to me, 'You're not to worry about your mum, the ambulance crew say she'll be fine when the doctors have finished with her. You're to stay with your grandfather.'

I stopped shaking. I wasn't warm and safe yet, but I knew I would be. I was going to Grandad's.

Inadvertently, I smiled. And became aware that John had been watching me. My eyes roved around the room. The invitations on the mantelpiece, the wall of books, the coal scuttle and small, neat pile of wood by the fire.

I swallowed. 'It's true that I did spend years in medical research thinking that I could maybe cure my mum's polio. When, obviously, I couldn't. Are you saying that now I'm moving into forensic psychiatry where the patients are violent because, well . . . because I subconsciously want to cure my dad?'

We both turned simultaneously to face each other, and simultaneously we laughed.

'Yes!' he said. And we laughed some more, although we weren't sure why.

John asked: 'Do you give a lot of thought to the victims of the patients you're dealing with? I sometimes wonder if it's better for us not to do that.'

'Yeah, I do find myself thinking about the victims,' I admitted, 'especially when they're children.'

'Duncan,' he began, seriously now, so seriously that I knew he had been waiting to say whatever came next. 'Have you thought of practising *child* forensic psychiatry?'

I looked at the fire through my whisky glass again. Its amber warmth was reflected in all directions.

He said: 'I have a gut feeling that you might move towards that. Your background might mean that you would come to it at a rather different angle from the rest of us.'

I had not thought of working with children, certainly not child offenders. Of course, I could never forget the first remarkable transformation I had seen in that ADHD child, what was his name, Benjamin? But I also remembered deciding, in the years straight after I qualified as a doctor, that paediatrics was not for me. In fact, perhaps because my childhood had been so difficult, I preferred not to deal with children at all. And, in my personal life, whenever a relationship began to look serious, I always warned the girlfriend that I did not want to have children of my own. So what on earth had given John the idea that I might decide to specialize in children, particularly child offenders? Probably because he himself had done that. I decided to respond diplomatically.

'The best thing about children for me is that they aren't so big and threatening as adults.'

He laughed. 'Oh, some children are very big and threatening! Duncan, you know, you can stop right now. You don't have to enter this world at all; you can simply drop crime and move to a safer place with safer patients.'

John Brontë was right, I didn't have to walk the dark, threatening alleys inside the minds of serious offenders. Except I did. I felt that I could not turn to right or left: my life was a path that had led me here and this was my destiny.

9

It is impossible to become a forensic psychiatrist without spending time in the high-security hospitals where offenders with severe and dangerous mental health problems are held. Many of the patients in these hospitals are psychopaths. By now I had assessed a number of psychopaths and I had developed a great interest in them.

Assessing a psychopath is often quite pleasant and interesting. That might be surprising when they, by definition, show a wholesale disregard for the rights or feelings of others: something all psychopaths have in common is a lack of empathy. But there are a number of other characteristics they may or may not share. They can be egotistical, easily bored, manipulative, untruthful, aggressive . . .

That sounds unattractive, and it certainly is. But it happens that many psychopaths are also charming, good talkers and entertaining company. I did very often notice a greatly inflated sense of entitlement, which seemed to be based on an assumption (and sometimes this assumption might have been correct), that they were the most intelligent person in the room. But that was the outer shell and I could never forget their core lack of empathy and callous disregard for suffering, including, perhaps especially, suffering they themselves had caused.

This liberation from empathy means that it tends to be psychopaths who commit our worst crimes. But, of course,

I was aware by now that there are plenty of psychopaths around who don't kill people or torture animals. They may live next door, they may be captains of industry, sports stars, perhaps even prime ministers. The psychopaths we were dealing with, however, all had criminal records. So what was the difference?

Maybe it was biological. But it was hard to ignore the fact that every criminal psychopath I met had a history which ticked a lot of boxes. Boxes for childhood deprivation, abuse, violence or neglect. Boxes for criminogenic or drug-abusing families.

Did that explain or excuse their offending?

For many of my colleagues, such a background went a long way to mitigating cruelty and crime. I simply could not share their view.

Most of the other psychiatrists had enjoyed quite comfortable childhoods – very different from the childhoods of the offenders they worked with. And, also, very different from mine. I am sure that family life for my colleagues was not perfect when they were young – all families have their complexities – but most of them acknowledged that they had been brought up by loving parents in a stable household with a stable income.

Maybe that explains why I saw things differently. I had been brought up amid cruelty, abuse and poverty. So I knew that a start like that was not good – but also that it did not necessarily lead to crime. And, as time went by, I became more and more sure that such a background did not excuse or mitigate violent criminality.

It was my interest in psychopathy that drove me towards some of the nation's most notorious offenders. When I started work at the high-security hospital, I recognized the names and even the faces of many patients from the news. But one of the very first patients I encountered was someone I recognized for another reason.

I'd been working at a big London hospital and shortly before I left had assessed a man for admittance to this same high-security hospital: his prison had feared that he was just too dangerous to be retained and wanted him moved. I had visited him in that prison and we had perched on benches in a concrete room facing each other. There was no one sitting next to me, but next to him were four officers, two on each side. To restrain him if necessary. And it was necessary.

'I do not want to go to a fucking mental hospital because there's nothing wrong with me and if you send me to a fucking mental hospital . . .' he said as he leapt as close to my face as he could with four officers jumping up behind to hold him back, '. . . I will find you out and I will do terrible things to your family. And you . . . as for you, I will kill you slowly, oh so slowly.'

Whoops, he had just got himself admitted to hospital. I did a full and thorough assessment, of course, and then referred him. He had next faced an admittance panel who, despite his angry protests, agreed with me that he was dangerous enough to become a high-security patient. And now here I was, on my first Saturday ward round.

I had assumed before I started work that patients would generally be in their cells. They were not. As a hospital, this was an open community. Patients were often milling about and today some were on their PlayStations, one group was playing cards and a few were watching TV.

'Make sure you add the eggs AFTER the butter,' instructed a TV chef. 'That's extremely important to maintain the right consistency.'

The men watching TV leaned forward. One nodded vigorously. Eggs after butter.

Several patients walked around in a purposeful way, although they were unlikely to have a purpose except perhaps to look at the new doctor out of the corner of their eyes. I had been asked to examine a facial wound which may have been self-inflicted and was making my way to the patient when a huge arm was clamped around my neck from behind.

I jumped and half turned. A man was towering over me, casually resting his hand across my shoulders now. It was the prisoner who had threatened to kill me slowly, oh so slowly, if I sent him to this very place.

'Doc!' he cried. 'Hey, Doc, how are you?'

I felt my heart pound, and as for that throb in my head which was still plaguing me, it became unbearable. Sweat broke out across my face. But now we had to pretend – that this was a normal meeting in a normal place under normal circumstances.

'Hey, good to see you! What are you doing today?' I asked.

'PlayStation!'

'Oh yeah, so what are you playing?'

'Wipeout,' he said. 'God, I love it.'

I had played a bit of Wipeout myself. We compared notes.

'It's the best racing game on the planet,' he assured me.

We went on to discuss other games. Actually, it was

quite an interesting discussion. So here we were, chatting as if we'd bumped into each other in the High Street. I was treating him like a human and not a murderer and serial offender, trying not to behave like a doctor who felt threatened by a seriously disordered and violent patient. Did I congratulate myself when we said a fond farewell and my heart resumed its normal rhythm? No, I did not, I was swamped by relief to find myself still alive.

Hospital was a better place for him to be and it was clear that now he knew that. He was on a rehabilitation ward where he was locked up for very few hours. I didn't say: 'I told you so.' Because it could so easily have gone the other way and, despite stringent safety procedures, this big man was quite capable of killing me in the seconds before help could arrive. I came off shift and went home to London that night with my head throbbing even more loudly than usual.

'It's so loud that I almost can't hear your voice,' I told my girlfriend as we made the dinner.

She walked across the kitchen to me and put her head close to mine and listened.

'It's funny,' she said. 'I sometimes think I can hear it throbbing.'

'My head? You can hear it throbbing inside?'

'Well . . . maybe not right now. But on the sofa when we were watching TV I thought I did. I must have been imagining it. And you're probably imagining it too. We both know that imagined symptoms feel real enough.'

'But if you think you can hear it –'

'I'm not sure . . .'

'I'm going to the doctor.'

We were both doctors, we both spent a lot of time inside heads, but we were the wrong sort of doctor.

'This is stress,' the GP said. 'You're working in a high-security hospital, you're exposing yourself to significant levels of danger every day. See what happens if you take a holiday.'

'But it's been going on a long time,' I told him. 'Through holidays too.' I suspected that it had started back when I had taken time out from doctoring and worked as a musician. I had gone back to medicine when I realized I wanted to be a psychiatrist, but by then I was enjoying music less. Now I wondered if the throb inside my head, distant then, had been the reason.

'I don't think it's anything to worry about,' the GP said.

I lived with my strange head condition for many more months before I returned to his surgery. I went back after something happened that caused an excessive amount of throbbing.

It was just a normal week. And a normal week in a high-security hospital might be spent with notorious serial killers.

I was having coffee with Alice.

'Sometimes I wonder what passes from these people to me,' I told her. 'I really fear a process of infusion. I ask myself if I'm absorbing something toxic.'

Alice was a nurse who had started work in the hospital at the same time as me. We had both gone through the long induction together where we'd learned self-defence manoeuvres and what to do if patients took us hostage. It was serious, but a lot of it made us laugh and by laughing together we'd become friends.

Beauty means different things to different people, but I think most would agree that Alice was beautiful, even when she looked hard at you and frowned, as now. She had a long neck, like a swan. When we chatted, she sometimes referred to a boyfriend. Lucky man.

She nodded slightly, waiting for me to say more. Something about Alice always made me want to say more.

'I do wonder about the way we have to collude with offenders to get the reports done, the way we spend time feeling real empathy for them and nodding our heads – just like you're nodding now.'

She smiled and stopped nodding, suddenly aware of herself.

'Alice, if we think about the victims, how can we do this job?'

'I couldn't do this job,' said Alice, 'if I didn't believe rehabilitation is possible for everyone.'

Her tone was confident. She looked down, arching her swan neck a little. 'My father was seriously alcoholic and made us all unhappy. No one thought there was any hope of him changing. But he did. One day he stopped drinking.'

My turn to nod empathically. 'Was he different after that?'

She gazed back, trusting me. Her eyes were green, flecked by brown.

'Unfortunately, he died about a year later.'

'Oh Alice, I'm sorry.'

'But it was a lovely year. I mean, all my life I'd seen glimpses of this kind, loving father. The man before the fourth drink. And now we had that man for a year. It was wonderful.'

She smiled. I smiled too.

'What was your dad like?' she asked.

'My dad could be nice,' I said quietly. 'But he wasn't always. I think he mellowed a bit as he got older.'

'There you are,' she said loudly, 'your dad changed too! Rehabilitation is always possible.'

It was true that, after my parents' divorce, my father had tried hard to be nicer. The judge said I should visit him every other Saturday and on those days we both pretended. Him to be a good father and me to be a good son.

'Late birthday present!' He handed me a cartoon book. 'You'll enjoy this, it's an adventure story.'

I sat down and started to read. And immediately I loved Tintin. He had a dog called Snowy and in the first few pictures Tintin and Snowy were walking down a country lane. The wind was blowing Tintin's coat. He strode out confidently, his face a strange mixture of young and old. He was unaware, or maybe he just didn't care, that he was wearing clothes which would draw a lot of comment in Guisborough.

He was going to see Captain Haddock. This was his friend, big and bearded and a bit scary, although Tintin had no fear because Captain Haddock took care of him. And together they had an amazing adventure.

The book was called *The Seven Crystal Balls* and I loved it.

Dad was first pleased and then annoyed when I couldn't stop reading.

'Let's go swimming,' he suggested.

At the pool, I said: 'You be Captain Haddock, and I'll be Tintin.'

That's who I wanted him to be. He, too, was big, hairy

and scary, so if he could be my Captain Haddock and come on adventures with me and take good care of me, everything would be all right. Because, despite the number of times he had hurt me and my mother or both of us, he was my dad and I loved him. But now Dad just looked helpless. He squinted at me with an air of hopelessness.

'What do you want me to do?'

'We're off on an adventure to discover the mysteries of Peru and you've got to chase me!'

Dad was embarrassed. And I was sad, because he probably wanted to play with me but he didn't know how. And how could he be Captain Haddock anyway when we both knew he might turn into a monster and beat me up without any warning?

I looked at him in the water and then looked rapidly away because it hurt so much to see him. Even when he tried very hard, he just wasn't good at being Dad.

Gradually, I visited him less often and eventually he didn't get in touch about the next visit, and neither did I, even though I was wracked with guilt by my own silence. The very last time I saw him was at a Working Men's Club. My band was playing and he had made a special effort to come. I was fourteen. I caught his eye from the stage and he gave me a thumbs-up and at that moment I realized that he wasn't a huge monster of a man but actually quite small. It was awkward, when we spoke briefly afterwards, to find that I was now taller than him. But I noticed that he seemed happier, calmer. He had a new family and, he said, a job he enjoyed. So maybe he really had changed.

Alice was smiling at me.

'See!'

I smiled back. I, like Alice, wanted to believe that rehabilitation was always possible. And I did believe it. Alice gave me more examples of people who had changed, her face slightly flushed, her voice energetic.

I remembered how I had never managed to persuade Joseph, the paedophile back in the Personality Disorder Unit, to feel empathy for his victims. But there were other forms of rehabilitation. And, anyway, I wanted to agree with Alice.

She had turned out to be an exceptional nurse. Firm, kind, compassionate. She played pool with the patients and often watched TV with them. I had seen a group of them talking about a programme with her once. The discussion was intense. I had written some reports, come back, and they were still there, still talking to her. Alice was always relaxed and she always saw the human behind the offender. She listened to their stories and laughed at their jokes and made them cups of tea. She was widely liked and, by me, admired. How did she always strike the right note? Training alone could not achieve that. She had either been born talented or she had learned from childhood how to manage people.

'These men are damaged and broken and we're here to help,' she said simply.

I had to agree. I was still the doctor who wanted to fix people. And Alice was inspiring.

I said: 'Recovery's an interesting word. I don't think we're likely to "cure" most of these men but –'

For a moment, Alice looked stubborn.

'We can do a lot for them!' she insisted.

'We know that most can never be let out of here. But

there's another way of defining recovery. If we try to give every patient the chance to aim for some sense of identity, purpose and social inclusion, that's a sort of recovery. I can give you a physical example to show what I mean. My mother's disabled, she contracted polio as a child . . .'

Alice's face crumpled into a picture of empathy. It made me feel good. All my life, people had jeered at my mother. She had experienced cruelty from strangers that I could not bear to remember, even now. But Alice wasn't like that. She looked as if she understood, as if she knew about the callipers and crutches and my mother's years of fighting to do what the able-bodied do.

I said: 'She's never going to recover from polio. That's impossible. But if cinemas have disabled access, if she can go out knowing there are toilets she can use, if she can travel on a train like everyone else, then that's a form of recovery.'

Alice agreed.

I said: 'Here's another example. I've been writing a report on Oscar: he's the college professor in this ward who killed his students. I've been talking to him about his life here . . .'

Her face lit up.

'I chat to Oscar quite often! He'd give anything to teach again. He loved teaching.'

'He loved teaching, but unfortunately he killed three students, so going back to college isn't a realistic option. But if we're driven by what the patient wants, by his skill set, and by what's realistic for him, then we can find a collaborative recovery pathway . . . for instance, he can teach some classes here, teach the other patients. That's a form of recovery, isn't it?'

We talked about this enthusiastically. I really believed in it. This was new thinking and I felt part of a new movement.

As we got up to return to our patients, Alice asked: 'How's your head these days?'

'No better. I've been to the GP but he's saying there's nothing wrong.'

Unlike everyone else, even my girlfriend, even my friends, even, yes, my mother, Alice didn't shrug and tell me that I was suffering from stress or some psychological symptom associated with my work.

'There must be a reason for this and your GP should be helping you find it,' she said wisely. 'I should go back to the surgery.'

A couple of mornings later, I crossed the television room and saw Alice there, wrapped up in *Bargain Hunt* with a small group of patients.

'I'm telling you, it's not even worth a fiver!' said a patient who had murdered four people and been locked up in hospital for years and years but was talking now as if he had popped into an auction house only last week.

Alice said: 'Oh, but it's very pretty.'

'Nah,' said another. 'That brooch is kitsch and I wouldn't bother to steal it.'

They all watched the screen intently to see what the brooch sold for.

'I bet it goes for more than twenty-five pounds,' said Alice as the bidding started. Everyone had an opinion on this. One person agreed with her but the others protested.

'No more than five!'

'All right, maybe ten, that's the max.'

'You'd have to be an idiot to pay more than ten.'

They were practically at the auction together. Alice's special skill.

Even I wanted to know how much the brooch fetched now. So I lingered nearby, watching the auction. I hardly noticed the patient approaching Alice from behind the sofa. If I did, I probably assumed he was joining the group. For a fraction of a second, I saw the flash of metal. And then the handle of the knife, wrapped in black masking tape. He was so close to her that for a moment I could do nothing but watch as he suddenly rounded the sofa and dug the blade into her right eye. I mean, fully into the eye, forcefully, with a hideous sound of penetration: of soft tissue, of vessels, of bone.

Blood exploded from Alice's eye socket. She screamed. A long, horrified, guttural scream of pain. Soon the blood was cascading down her face, spraying across the room. One of the men, the one who thought the brooch was worth ten pounds and no more, grabbed her assailant and held him with an arm across his throat.

The weapon was still sticking out of Alice's eye like the most unfunny cartoon ever. She thrashed uncontrollably on the sofa. At first, I was frozen with horror and the only thing that moved was the big throb inside my head. Then I was at her side, trying to hold her while her body jerked dangerously near the edge of the sofa in a seizure.

A nurse rushed up and stretched towards the weapon to pull it out.

‘Leave it,’ I said. ‘Or you could cause more damage. Call an ambulance!’

The nurse stepped back and stared at Alice. He, too, had frozen.

‘Call an ambulance,’ I repeated, surprised at how loud and clear my voice was. He turned and ran from the room, nearly tripping over the response team, who had arrived and were now restraining the assailant on the floor behind the sofa.

Chaos. Medics. Equipment. People everywhere, in the room, shouting in the hallway. The crash team alarm ringing, another alarm too – or was that inside my head? And, the blood. I was holding Alice, muttering words that I hoped were comforting, when a patient came up close.

‘I need my medication, Doc, I need it right now, give me my medication, Doc, Doc, I must have it, Doc . . .’

He was yelling in my ear, across the bloody mess that was Alice. He would not stop. I knew this was the last thing Alice needed. She was still now but the blood was flowing out of her eye socket like a spring which would never dry. I moved aside to deal with the selfish, demanding patient as the medical team took over. I tried to forgive him – I knew Alice would have. She would have understood that he was sick and couldn't help it, that his desperate expression of some need, any need, was his way of dealing with Alice's immense need.

The ambulance arrived and she was stabilized. She lay on a stretcher, head back, her neck looking impossibly long as she was carried out. A wounded swan. At the hospital she went straight into trauma surgery. Later we learned that her eye had been completely eviscerated and the oculoplastic surgeons who were called in from a specialist centre had removed it.

When I tried to visit her in hospital, I was told that she did not want to see anyone from work. I wasn't surprised. And I doubted that this effortlessly brilliant nurse would ever find herself on a ward with patients again. As for her assailant, he had carefully hand-made the knife for his attack using some metal he'd somehow extracted from a cupboard-door mechanism. The operation had been planned in detail. But he could give no reason why.

Alice wasn't the only person to leave the high-security hospital after the attack. I didn't stay much longer. The throbbing in my head had become so violent that it was hard to live with and I felt the stress of working with such high-security patients might be exacerbating the problem, whatever the problem was. Besides, a friend and mentor, Ari Good, had lots of work lined up for me in London.

10

I made further attempts to contact Alice but I did not succeed. I still wonder what happened to her. I hope that she returned to nursing, perhaps in a safer environment. Had the attack stopped stone dead her passion for believing in others and helping them? I could not find out.

I did, however, follow the advice she had given me. I took my loud, throbbing head back to my GP. This time he not only referred me for a CT scan but also to a tinnitus clinic. I had the scan and then waited. Weeks passed. No news. It seemed they were going to make me wait forever. Or maybe they had found precisely nothing and weren't bothering to inform me.

One summer Saturday I was sitting at my desk at home trying to get some work done. As usual, the big drum banging in my head was competing for space with my thoughts. Today, it was winning. I sighed and stopped work. Dr Who and Tintin stared down at me from their shelf. My eye ran over the familiar contours of these old friends. As a kid, I didn't know which one I loved most. Dr Who was the man I wished would be my father. But it was my real father who had brought Tintin into my life and sometimes Tintin felt like all that was left of him.

'Duncan, are you talking to Tintin, for God's sake?' asked my girlfriend sharply, appearing in the doorway. Her eyes were narrowed, her tone was beady. She did not like my relationship with things I regarded as precious and she regarded as toys.

'Yes,' I said. 'He's an old mate and we often have a chat.'

'Well, stop that, because it's a lovely day. Let's go down to the river.'

I was surprised. This wasn't her usual sort of excursion. But as soon as we reached the river, I was glad we'd come here. The sun was a blister in the sky and the river world was green and lush and luxuriant. I often felt agitated these days, but the river was calming. Its flow was even and unchanging – never faster, never slower. I closed my eyes and the sun's heat fell on the back of my head. Its river reflection warmed my face, my eyelids. In retrospect, it seems to me that for a few seconds the hammer in my head didn't bang quite so hard. That my world was full of hope.

When I opened my eyes, my girlfriend was watching me.

She said: 'You've got a brain tumour.'

I blinked.

And, in that fraction of a second while I blinked, the whole world changed. The river was still there, the grass, the heavy summer trees. It all looked the same. But it was different because I was different.

This moment took place some years ago but I've never been that man again, the man who shut his eyes in the sun by the river. He was always sustained by hope, a deep belief that, as my grandfather often said, things would be all right. Now, suddenly, as if the tide had gone out, all hope was drained. The man by the river had disappeared.

She said: 'It was so weird that they haven't given you the

scan result. I guessed it must have got lost in the system. That's why I asked Jamie to access it.'

Jamie was one of her best mates, a registrar at the hospital where I'd been scanned.

'So. Listen up. I've got the scan report and it's a brain tumour.'

I opened my mouth but no words came out.

'They think it's a glomus jugulare.'

This meant nothing to me.

'It's not looking good, I'm afraid. I had to do quite a bit of research because it's so rare. But, basically, when other people can hear your head throbbing, that's one of the most recognizable symptoms. You'll need brain surgery and it's risky, of course. There's one good thing though: the cancer's unlikely to have spread.'

I might have wondered how she broke bad news to her patients if she broke bad news to her partner this way. But that only occurred to me later. Right now, I was hardly able to process the information: it took me not hours but days to do that, perhaps weeks. And, finally, I understood that Dr Harding had become a patient. An educational experience for any doctor.

It took further weeks to persuade the hospital that they had missed the scan report and should see me. At last I found myself in the office of an eminent professor, a brain tumour specialist and no stranger to the fascinating phenomenon that was glomus jugulare. I liked him at once. He was very large and bearded and he looked like Captain Haddock.

He scrutinized his screen and shook his grizzled head.

'This tumour is strange. It's so vascular. That's not unusual, of course, but in your case it's unusually vascular. We'll have to investigate further before I can think of operating.'

Many tumours are sustained by the blood vessels which carry them the nutrients they need to grow and spread until they kill us. So mine was unusually vascular. I was sure that was not good.

'Er . . . operating?' I echoed faintly.

'I can't pretend it will be a safe operation. I'll have to go through some cranial nerves on the left side of your head, obviously, and the results of that could be deafness, palsy, stroke . . .'

By the time I left, I had only absorbed two facts: that I would die if he did not operate and be disabled if he did.

It was hard to concentrate on anything between the mosaic of scans I now faced: MRIs, CTs, MRIs with contrast, CTs with contrast . . . but I did try to keep working and my colleague Ari Good was ready to give me plenty of cases. My mind flipped around like a fish out of water. I wanted to learn a lot more about forensic psychiatry. It was a journey and I had far to travel. But what was the point if I was going to die?

For now I decided to indulge the interest I had developed in psychopaths. If anything could keep me focused and absorbed, it would be psychopathy. Something about extreme disorders was simple and primitive when I was becoming simple and primitive and disordered myself. I was focusing more and more on my own needs, on my fears and on my tumour in a narcissistic way that some people label 'survival narcissism'.

As I ricocheted between scanners, I distracted myself by falling back into research. It was like putting on some comfortable and well-worn clothes. This time, the research was into psychopathy and it actually took me to more scanners. We plucked eight psychopaths from medium-secure units and scanned their brains. I offered to pay them each £50 for this.

Some could not resist a try-on.

'Er, the doctor said we were being paid a hundred pounds, yes, that's what he definitely told us,' they claimed (unsuccessfully) when they arrived, handcuffed, at the scanner unit.

The results of our research were never published: our sample was too small and further work was necessary. I did not want to do that work. Why should I care about it, I asked myself, if I was going to die anyway?

My belief in my imminent demise meant I took on no cases of my own. But I did grow in this long period. Ari Good was one of a team of forensic psychiatrists working at a big London hospital and I became immersed in some of their cases.

Our role as forensic psychiatrists within the criminal justice system was often to answer a straightforward question: is this defendant mentally fit to plead? Some people are so ill or so impaired that they simply cannot understand their own plea, or what is going on in court, or they are not well enough to play an active part in it.

Our second role was to assess the defendant for the defence or prosecution. We wrote reports on the mental state of the defendant, if and when they had committed the crime. And we had to be ready to defend our conclusions in court.

'As soon as you're well enough, you'll get some big cases coming your way,' Ari Good said in a kind voice. 'You're ready.'

He was tall and thin and wrinkly and when he smiled his wrinkles all rearranged themselves around his mouth so that his whole face smiled.

I nodded and said nothing. Because I was a man with no future.

Ari studied me.

'Want to go on the witness stand for Jimmy Phipp?' he asked, as if enticing a sick child to eat. We enjoyed discussing Jimmy Phipp. He illustrated all our differences.

'No,' I said. 'I don't want to defend him. I think he killed knowing exactly what he was doing and I think he's really dangerous.'

We all privately reach our own conclusions and those were mine, even though it was of course the jury's job to decide if Phipp was guilty of murder.

He was accused of killing his business and sexual partner, Carlo Spagnola. Carlo's body had been found, cut into pieces, in Jimmy's freezer and every shred of evidence said that Jimmy had put it there. Phipp had initially denied all knowledge of the homicide, behaving aggressively to his defence team and suggesting to the police that some mysterious stranger from Carlo's past must be responsible. He had even invented that past: the killer was an avenging mafioso from Calabria. He made it sound plausible, even though Carlo came not from Calabria in the south but from the mountains of northern Italy.

The problem with this scenario was that the avenging mafioso had managed to kill Spagnola without leaving any

DNA whatsoever. But traces of Phipp were found everywhere – not just on the body, but on the bag into which Carlo had been stuffed. Fibres and fingerprints combined with incriminating phone messages to make this look like a textbook case. Phipp had a string of convictions for violence and had been suspected of murder before. But this was the first time there had been such strong evidence against him.

At the last minute, Jimmy Phipp agreed to change his plea to guilty. Not to murder, but to manslaughter. That is when Ari and I were brought in. Had he killed Spagnola because he was mentally ill?

We interviewed him extensively and agreed that he was a psychopath: he was incapable of experiencing pain or regret for any of the suffering he caused others. The horrible death of his friend and business associate left him unmoved. He was more worried about contamination to his freezer, which contained small wooden objects he was treating for woodworm – Phipp was an antiques trader.

'I wouldn't buy a Georgian card table from him,' Ari admitted. 'The legs would certainly turn out to be made of plywood.'

'And I wouldn't defend him on a murder charge,' I said. Psychopathy is not regarded as mitigation and is not a defence.

Ari laughed. 'Oh, that's quite different.'

Phipp was pleading diminished responsibility and we were to help the defence prove that his mental functioning meant he was not responsible for his actions.

Anyone who successfully pleads diminished responsibility is telling the court that they are ill and so should, of course, on sentencing, usually be admitted to a secure hospital, not prison. There the patient should be assessed and, if possible, treated. That is the psychiatrist's point of view. But my worry was that, as far as offenders and their lawyers are concerned, manslaughter with diminished responsibility might very often mean just one thing: a chance of earlier release.

This perhaps makes manslaughter with diminished responsibility an attractive plea and it also makes psychiatrists who will confirm the existence of a mental health condition much in demand. Since all scientific facts are open to interpretation, it is usually possible to find some psychiatrist, somewhere, who will interpret the facts in favour of the defence. Ari Good, a decent, kind and well-meaning man, could usually be relied upon to help the defence.

'I've told you, I don't remember nothing about what happened,' Phipp said. He had drained a paper cup of water and was now throwing it up in the air and catching it adeptly. He was not the sort of psychopath who made us laugh.

'Carlo comes over my place, we have a few drinks and a bit of fun and we fall asleep. I wake up with something cold and horrible beside me and it's Carlo. I panicked then, I was scared someone would think I'd killed him. I was scared I *had* killed him. I didn't know what I was doing when I cut him up, it was blind panic did that, not me.'

He threw the cup in the air. There was a moment when we both expected him to drop it. We watched in silence. He caught it.

'You woke up and found him dead – do you have any

memory of holding the knife, of stabbing him with it?' asked Ari with great tenderness, as if talking to a lost child.

Jimmy Phipp shrugged and waved the cup with an air of helplessness. He was a very thin man and his shoulder bones protruded through his clothes.

'Had a few drinks, that's all I remember. Doc, are you going to get me out of here? I hate jail, I get so depressed.'

I found myself thinking that one way to avoid getting depressed in jail would be to stop committing violent crimes, but that seemed not to have occurred to Jimmy Phipp. When he talked about his depression he blamed it on the prison officers, the other inmates and his parents.

Ari was far more sympathetic to this than I could be.

'Just think of Jimmy Phipp's childhood,' he reminded me later, his wrinkles etching tragedy on his face. 'It's hardly surprising he grew up with mental health challenges.'

'The jury isn't going to let him off because he's a psychopath,' I said.

Ari winced, as though in pain. 'Oh, but didn't he tell us how he suffers terribly in jail from bouts of mood disorder with depression? You know how he was on suicide watch throughout his last sentence.'

'Yes, he told us all about that. But isn't it interesting that he doesn't seem to connect the sound of a siren rushing towards his bloodied victims with a prison sentence and his subsequent depression?'

'For heaven's sake, Duncan, where is your compassion? He was six when his father tried to drown him in the sea at Clacton! His mother drank herself to death. He witnessed abuse in the family on a daily basis, and if he didn't witness it, he received it. How can we be surprised if Jimmy Phipp grew up with depressive episodes which contribute to his violence?'

'He needs help,' I agreed. 'Although the chances of changing a fifty-seven-year-old psychopath are slim.'

Slim, but I still believed that, even for Jimmy, change might be possible. I wondered what Alice would have made of him. Had her core belief, that rehabilitation was possible for everyone, really endured? I had tried again to contact her, without success.

I could not share her views now, but I wanted to think that it was possible for some people to change. Believing that brought hope to our work.

'With treatment,' I said, 'perhaps Jimmy can learn to deal with his past in other, non-violent ways. But he should be kept locked up a long time for public safety until he's addressed that and learned about violence reduction. He shouldn't be let out to hurt someone else by a group of professionals saying it's really not his fault.'

Ari's face fell dramatically, all his wrinkles sagging south.

I said: 'I am absolutely sure that Jimmy intended to stab Carlo. He finally admitted there had been a row.'

Intent can be the difference between murder and manslaughter. So I was surprised when Ari nodded vigorous agreement.

'Certainly, Jimmy is a psychopath and intended to kill Carlo,' he cried. 'But he was also suffering from an appalling mood disorder at the time, he was deeply depressed, and this meant he was unable to control his actions. Can't you see that, Duncan?'

At Jimmy Phipp's trial, Ari's handwringing and his busy wrinkles seemed to work their magic on the jurors. At least half looked deeply moved and a few threw Phipp glances of great compassion. When we broke for them to reach their verdict, the defence was confident. But, to everyone's surprise, it took the jury just a couple of hours to find him guilty of murder and not manslaughter. There was wailing and clapping in the public gallery from the respective families of Jimmy and Carlo. Jimmy scowled darkly at his defence team, as if we, and not he, were responsible for his jail sentence.

'We have simply no way of telling what a jury's going to do,' said Ari in the pub afterwards. The defence team stared down at their drinks and shook their heads in agreement.

The barrister looked morose. 'I really thought we'd get manslaughter with diminished.'

They were sad because they had failed to reduce Jimmy's sentence by convincing the jury that Jimmy just couldn't help stabbing Carlo and that a bit of medication would make him safe for release. But deep down, they knew this was not true. He had been nasty and dangerous even to members of his own defence team: a couple of juniors had been threatened. If the jury had agreed that Phipp's crime was caused by depression, then he could simply have been given anti-depressants and all too soon released on to the streets. Even if he was still nasty and dangerous.

Ari Good lived up to his name: he was a good man and a good doctor and I admired him as a forensic expert. But I did not agree with him that, at its heart, crime always stems from some mental disorder. For him, cruelty could not be part of human behaviour, it had to be an illness.

Perhaps believing that cruelty could be understood and treated with compassion and care allowed him to do his job, to carry on as the good doctor day after day. Perhaps my father was mentally ill and, with his own good doctor, he might not have hurt his small son. Perhaps.

Personally, I was relieved that Jimmy had been convicted of murder. I decided then and there that, if I lived to work as a forensic psychiatrist, I would be objective and truthful and not defend the indefensible. I thought I could still be a good doctor without assuming that cruelty could be medicalized and treated away. A priority must be to prevent offenders from claiming further victims. Because if I played a role in the exoneration or early release of someone dangerous who then went on to hurt someone else, I knew I would have to accept some responsibility. Not in law. But in my heart.

11

Eventually, I was back in the hospital to hear the professor's conclusions after all those scans. I sat down swamped by fear and misery and a sort of nothingness, a void for him to fill with the news that I would soon die.

'Sorry,' he said. 'I realize this is very frustrating for you. We have a confusing picture. So I've booked you in for a PET scan.'

In the radiology waiting room, I couldn't help noticing that all the other patients were elderly. They sat meekly, not looking at anything. Was this how sheep behave at the slaughterhouse? I did not want to be a sheep and accept my fate meekly. I wanted to leap from my seat and argue with someone. When I was led into a darkened room and radioactive substances were injected into my veins, I felt frightened and angry and invaded instead of grateful for the wonders of modern medicine. When I was put into a tube and scanned, I wanted to wriggle free, shouting. It's true that doctors make terrible patients.

There were two weeks to wait for the results and those two weeks were hard.

'Got a very interesting homicide case, the defendant just can't stop strangling women!' said Ari in a tone of enticement. But I did not respond. Even my fascination with the criminal mind failed me now.

I tried to retreat to a place of solace I had first turned to long ago. Music. But now my enjoyment of music, of the guitar, was impaired by the thudding in my brain. Which was never in time with the music.

If music couldn't save me then nothing would, and I grew quieter and sadder until hope disappeared and the world became an ugly, pointless void. I don't present myself to patients as a man with lived experience of severe mental health problems, but that period of my life gave me more than a glimpse of the darkness.

Then an email arrived from the professor.

> *Duncan, I wanted to let you know at once. The entire scan is NEGATIVE. There is no evidence of a primary tumour and no evidence of a secondary. Further investigation necessary.*

My first feeling was relief. My second was disbelief. Further investigation was necessary because, obviously, something was very wrong.

The next day I saw the professor. He stroked his beard.

'I am finding your results extremely perplexing. What we're seeing is so vascular in nature. Obviously, we've been assuming that this is an above normal vascularity in a tumour, but we can't find the tumour. However, I can't rule it out completely until you've had a cranial angiogram.'

This was a neurosurgical procedure, with all its risks.

'I'd like sedation, please,' I told the neurosurgeon.

She smiled.

'Sorry, we can't do that. We need to check you throughout the surgery to make sure you're not having a stroke and for that we need you wide awake, not sedated.'

She passed me a consent form.

'What are the chances of a stroke?'

She looked evasive. Then said: 'There's a small chance of a major complication like that. I'm sorry. And perhaps I should warn you that we include death in the list of major complications.'

It wasn't long before I was lying on a metal table, fully awake, while people in masks leaned over me. I was starring in my own horror movie. They made an incision into my femoral artery and it was painful. I was aware of the insertion of a wire. Up my leg, through my heart, up, up through my body. I felt the hot dye go in. It was burning the back of my eyeballs as it diffused into my brain.

I thought that being a patient in an operation was like being a psychiatrist. My job was to receive. To receive crime, to hear all the monstrous things patients told me they had done, to regard with humanity other men's inhumanity. And what could I feel now, creeping through my brain? To me it seemed that it was all the poison I had absorbed from patients.

When they removed the wire from my body, my femoral artery wouldn't stop bleeding; I was admitted overnight. Bandaged, bloody and bruised, I was released the next morning to the waiting professor.

'I was sure it couldn't be a tumour, but I hardly knew what else it could be except a fistula,' he said. 'Although a complex cluster of dural arteriovenous fistulas like yours is extraordinarily rare. And so very fascinating!'

I sighed. I know it is never good to fascinate doctors.

He leaned forward. He placed his large, bearded Captain Haddock chin on his fingers. His elbows rested on the desk.

'Was there some sort of an accident long ago, when you were a child?' he asked.

I thought hard.

'I don't think so.'

'How about a head injury?

'I can't remember anything . . .'

'An accident, perhaps, which caused a severe blow to the head?'

I had taken plenty of blows to the head, some of them severe, but they weren't accidents. I didn't want to tell the professor about my father so I looked vague and he evidently decided not to pursue his questions.

'These fistulas can arise for no apparent reason but, looking at all the scans, it's clear that, some time earlier in life, for some reason, you developed a very large blood clot in your cavernous sinus. As a result, many tiny arteries formed in that area so that your blood could navigate its way around the blockage. You've had it a long time now and of course the fistula has grown bigger and bigger until it looks like a ball of wool, a very ragged ball.'

It felt more like wire than wool. Barbed wire. Right now, as usual, it was throbbing in time with my heart.

'How can you treat it?' I asked.

He did not look at me. His eyes wandered to the window. Outside in the street were voices; young people, students perhaps, chattering away in many different languages. I heard their vigour, their youth, their energy. Death was distant for them.

'Well, your neurosurgeon feels that there is no safe treatment.'

'No treatment! You mean I have to live like this?'

He looked startled. Had I raised my voice?

'Duncan, we'll take some other views as well. I've had a preliminary chat with someone at Queen Square and they were more sanguine. We need to look into the options and the risks.'

I had worked at Queen Square in my medical research days. It is neurology's epicentre in the UK.

'What are the risks of doing nothing?'

'It could burst. Causing stroke, seizures or death, I'm afraid.'

'There must be treatment!'

'I'm going to discuss this. You'll have to give me time.'

I tried not to look impatient.

'Just go back to work. Get on with your life,' the professor advised me. 'I know how hard it must be with so many tiny arteries screaming in your ear every time your heart beats. But try to look outwards and ignore it if you can, because there really may be no treatment.'

Ignore it? Impossible. Live with it? Also impossible.

When I went back to work, I was feeling very angry. This was all my father's fault. I shut my eyes and I was four years old as he picked me up off the garden path by my T-shirt, roaring because my toy cars were making a mess in the gravel. I saw his fist, a wavy line on its horizon. Thick with fingers. Then my face cracked open into a thousand small pieces of pain like shattered glass. I shut my eyes.

'Fucking little shit, making a mess out here!'

I lolled forward, a puppet with its string broken. But I knew he was making another fist. He pulled up my face and . . . smash. This time all the small fragments of pain became one big pain. If all the trees were one tree, what a great tree that would be. If all the seas were one sea . . . My mother had taught me the poem and now, as my head swelled and then shattered, I thought: if all the pain was one pain, what a great pain that would be.

As an adult, I understood that his punches were more than painful: they were toxic. He had hit a young boy so often that he had poisoned that boy's adulthood. Here was a man who believed that his own adulthood had been poisoned by his father: didn't he always say that his epilepsy had been caused because his father hit him so hard? So why had he done the same to me?

We were physical proof that all parents scar as well as nurture their children. The mental damage may endure but usually the physical damage heals. Not in my father's case, not in mine: the physical consequences had simply worsened.

My mother was thrilled by the news that I was tumour-free.

'Oh Duncan, I wish your father was alive so you could tell him the trouble he caused with his violence!' she cried. 'But anyway, thank heavens it'll be all right now.'

Everyone at work also thought it would be all right now. I should take on cases of my own and generally act like a man with a future, they insisted. My head throbbed just as insistently as ever while they told me how pleased they were.

'This is wonderful!' beamed Ari. 'There's no tumour. And you're back just in time for such an interesting case! The one I told you about, the man who can't stop strangling women. His name's Jonathan Bowyer and the prosecution want you to be their expert witness.'

Ari did not want to handle Jonathan Bowyer's case himself because he really did not like working for the prosecution. He nearly always found a way to construct a psychiatric defence because he hated to put people away. Even murderers.

'If forensic psychiatry is about the interface between criminal justice and mental health, there is no better place to find out about it than on the witness stand at the Old Bailey,' he told me cheerfully. It sounded like one of his lectures to students.

Giving evidence in a headline-grabbing trial at the Old Bailey was going to be a challenge. Especially with a large ball of barbed wire throbbing inside my head.

Colleagues were not so optimistic as Ari.

'The defence will be a top silk and they'll give you hell on the stand,' they said, gloomily. They all could, and did, tell me stories of systematic attempts by foxy barristers to undermine their credibility and professionalism in the witness box.

'No, no, no,' countered Ari. 'Facing stringency in court is good for us. It's an excellent opportunity to examine our approaches, our actions, our thoughts.'

The colleagues gave him withering looks. They believed we should do all that – but in team meetings, not in front of a judge and jury.

They regarded me with compassion. 'Good luck with this one!' they said kindly.

12

I set off for jail to meet Jonathan. Prisons were becoming a way of life now. At first I had been intimidated by them: the even tread of the prison officers who led me down long, echoing corridors, the constant jangling of keys, the strange rhythm of doors, one after another, opening before us and clanging behind us. Why would anyone sacrifice fresh air for this?

Gradually, though, I got used to prisons, the way inmates do. Each one is different and each one is the same.

I had not visited Jonathan's prison before and the sat nav took me to a dead end. I turned around and drove up long streets lined by terraced houses, the prison's towering walls always in view but its entrance elusive. The houses seemed faceless, or perhaps it was that they preferred not to look. I wondered what it was like living with a view of such unrelenting and solid brick, topped by rolls of barbed wire.

As usual, there was nowhere to park. The locals had ensured prison business never found its way on to their streets. And the car park itself was packed, the space I'd reserved nearly impossible to find.

Footsteps, keys, doors. Eventually I arrived in the room where Jonathan waited. He was the size of a truck. I am tall but it would have taken a man of his bulk just a few seconds to strangle me. So when I heard the prison officer's footsteps retreating outside, I hoped he was staying within earshot.

But Jonathan turned out to be surprisingly genial.

'Hello, mate!' he said cheerfully.

I explained why I was here and we chatted about prison food: Jonathan had been working in the kitchen. By the time he had signed my consent form, I had understood that here was an amiable, even charismatic man. It wasn't that he was telling me jokes, but he was nevertheless humorous.

'This isn't your first time in prison,' I said.

'Nah, did a stretch for robbery a few years back. Did the crime, paid the time and that was me and robbery over and done with. Hardly made a penny from it anyway.'

'Who did you rob?' I asked. He had been an office cleaner in the City of London; surely there were plenty of chances to steal then from wealthy traders. He had also worked as a nightclub bouncer. But he said he had never stolen from his place of work.

'Nah, not worth the risk. I did nursing homes. Have you seen those places, mate? Ever been in one?'

I shook my head.

'Well, talk about the life of fucking Riley. Comfy chairs, radiators on max, old dears bringing you a cuppa and a good-sized slice of Victoria sponge. I tell you, mate, when I retire that's where I want to go and if you've any sense you'll do the same.'

'What did you steal?'

'Rich pickings there, fucking rich pickings. Jewellery, money, little trinkets made of solid silver that they've had in the family since time began. But I never made much out of it really. Didn't have the contacts to get me what the stuff was worth.'

Jonathan was fascinating. His face wove itself into interesting shapes as he spoke; fleeting smiles became wide-eyed wonder became a matey half-wink.

'How did you get caught?'

'I was too breezy, that was the trouble. Don't ever, ever relax, that's how you get collared – but I'd done the place before and thought I knew all about it. So one day I wanted a new television: old one was crap. I know this place and I'm sure I remember where all the cameras are and I take them all out. Except I didn't. I fucking missed one! I've only gone and given them a shot of my ugly mug! But I don't know that, so I park right outside and jimmy a window. Don't even need to be quiet, they're all deaf as posts in there. Then my usual routine: pull out some bacon and eggs and make a nice fry-up. See, people smell that, or they come downstairs and see someone in the kitchen, and they think you must be staff.'

I looked impressed.

'I just told you a trick of the trade there, mate,' he chuckled. 'Works every time, try it!'

I found myself chuckling too.

'Anyway, they've got a lounge with a nice big telly, and I mean it's a fifty incher, and it was absolutely fucking heavy. "Oh, let me help you," says some old geezer, tottering over to me. Holds open the door . . .' He was laughing now. 'Even follows me and holds the van door open. So home I goes and I don't think much more about it. I've got the telly in time to watch Chelsea smash Arsenal, but the game's no sooner begun than there's a knock on the door.

It's Old Bill! Most of them aren't gifted with brains but they don't have to be because, fuck me, the TV's right in front of their eyes showing blokes in shorts running around Stamford Bridge.'

He transformed his face into an archetypal police officer's, a stern-voiced, unsmiling pillar of justice.

'"Can you tell me where you acquired that television, Mr Bowyer?"'

We both laughed. I asked him about his childhood, his physical health, about being a cleaner and a nightclub bouncer.

'So, being a bouncer: it's all about fucking diplomacy, see,' he said. 'I should work for the fucking Foreign Office. Of course, if difficult punters don't like that, there are other ways of dealing with them.'

Did cruelty flicker across his ever-changing face? Did I catch it for a fraction of a second? I wasn't sure. I did know that anyone in jail accused of murder is going to be wearing a mask and that it was my job to see behind that mask. So I had to watch Jonathan like a hawk, catch any glimpses I could of his changing presentation and then, as far as possible, unpack what I'd seen.

I asked about his psychiatric history, his use of drugs, his criminal record. I was making notes as he talked because I knew the court might ask to see these. And at the same time, I was watching to see if the mask slipped, trying to register every tiny twitch, every nuance of non-verbal communication. This was particularly hard because Jonathan bombarded me with nuances. His expressions, his hand movements, his busy eyebrows, his constantly twisting mouth: looking for the real Jonathan underneath it all was like peering through a windscreen covered in flies.

Finally we arrived at an important point in the interview. It was time to ask about his relationships. We were edging nearer now to discussing the index offence. Jonathan was accused of murdering his wife. She was not his first wife. There had been many relationships. And he had been charged six times in the past with assault. Six different women had accused him of strangling them seriously enough to bring charges. However, he had never been convicted.

'I've seen some reports about allegations from previous partners. We don't need to speak about that now, but I wondered if there's anything you want to say about it?'

Jonathan shrugged, looking away. There was nothing he wanted to say about it now or ever. His face was still, giving me a brief chance to study him in repose. He looked angry and discontented: I hadn't seen this face until now. Was this what lay behind the mask?

'We do need to speak about what happened with your wife, though. I know it's not easy, but can you tell me what happened that night?'

His presentation changed again. He looked reflective, thoughtful, then upset, genuinely upset.

'She just did my head in,' he said. 'Simple as. Yap, yap fucking yap.'

'What were you talking about that night?'

Without hesitation, he said: 'Tiling. Tile this, tile that. Always the same thing. She knows I can't tile, she knows I hate it, but oh no, she has to have the fucking bathroom retiled. I wish I never painted it. If I hadn't changed the colour of the walls, she wouldn't have wanted the colour of the tiles changed. But she was obsessed. Life could not go on unless the bathroom tiles were changed. Yap, yap, yap.'

He shook his head. He was distressed now. And I couldn't help suspecting that it was the tiling and not the death of his wife that was causing this distress.

'What happened next?'

'I just lost it, Doc.' He clenched his fists. 'On and on and on she goes until . . .' He stopped abruptly. 'Next thing, she was quiet as a church mouse, laying there in bed like she was still asleep and the tiling didn't matter no more.'

I waited for him to continue. He didn't. He sat looking down at his huge fingers.

'Do you remember what happened?' I asked at last.

'Nah, mate. It's just all blank.'

'What about afterwards?'

He shrugged and remained silent. So now Jonathan wasn't talking and even attempts by me to ask him about the nursing home burglaries didn't persuade him to speak again.

At the main door I was greeted by the wind, buffeting me gently. Rain pattered as I threaded my way through the densely parked cars, and rain had never felt so good. There is always a certain joy in leaving a prison, even if you aren't an inmate.

Jonathan was dangerous, I knew that. This was indicated by his immediate command of the interview, the engaging personality he could switch on or off. His denial of responsibility. The lapse into silence when met with questions about the offence or those previous charges. His apparent inability to feel any compassion for his dead wife. His lack of regret.

He was dangerous but I did not think he was mentally ill. After careful questioning, I could find no evidence of a health condition that would explain or excuse Jonathan's loss of control when he strangled his wife. Anger, of course, is not mental illness.

I wrote a report for the prosecution confirming that there was no clinical condition to suggest this was manslaughter and not murder. Privately, I thought that being married to him must have been a roller coaster for his wife. How could she know who was coming home? The charmer, the silent husband, or the menacing stranger?

And there was an extra element to this case. I had attempted to ask Jonathan about it, but he had maintained his silence.

His wife had entered the marriage from a previous relationship, and she had brought with her a child. Jonathan's stepdaughter was called Jessica and she was eight years old when her mother died. She had been in her room, hiding in a cupboard, while Mrs Bowyer was killed. Perhaps Jonathan had forgotten she was there, perhaps he didn't care.

He had taken his wife's body into the bathroom. Here, he had wrapped her in black plastic. Then he had left the flat for good – in fact he had gone to Portugal, where he was later arrested.

A neighbour had heard enough to call the police and Jessica was found clinging to the partially unwrapped body of her mother. She refused to leave and had finally been dragged away, screaming. And this was what I found most upsetting about the case. The huge, violent Jonathan and a woman's body wrapped in plastic was bad enough. But worst of all was the small girl bent over the body, screaming, traumatized for life. I should have been thinking about Jonathan. But it was Jessica I could not get out of my mind.

13

The prosecution accepted my report and I waited for Jonathan's trial, which was scheduled to take place months hence. But before the date came around, something amazing happened.

The thundering in my ear, night and day, had robbed me of sleep. It had stopped me reading. And it had come between me and music, one of my most important relationships. There were days when work was impossible. I dreaded appearing at the Old Bailey for Jonathan's trial with such a handicap. I disclosed my health condition to the court but, having established that it did not affect my cognition, they were happy to proceed. Then suddenly the professor contacted me to say he had found a doctor who was confident that he could operate successfully on my ball of throbbing barbed wire.

So I went into hospital for an operation. It was fraught with risk. Over many hours, the surgeon managed to block the knot of tiny arteries in my head with a combination of metal coils and glue, while keeping the important vessels functioning.

I woke up to silence. An absence of noise so intense that it was more like a vacuum. A hole in my head. A missing limb.

The vacuum was filled, briefly, by anger. I had gone through all this because a man who was supposed to love and protect me had punched me hard and often. And, although I was cured for now, the professor had warned me that the problem might recur in future years. My working life had been built on the premise that the mind – as well as the body – of every adult tells the story of their childhood, and now this had been brutally illustrated in a most personal way.

That adults make decisions with long-term consequences for us when we are young was certainly not news to me. That they nurture us and damage us and we live with the effects of this even when we are old – this was not news either. That it was hard or even impossible to save adults from damage inflicted long ago was a conclusion I was reaching. And I now understood that the best chance of reversing damage must be during childhood.

Lying in my hospital bed, I came to a decision even I had not expected. Obviously, to make a real difference, I must work with children. No one had helped me when my father had attacked me. Someone should have helped, all children should be helped. Before it's too late.

Over the next days, weeks, even months, there was a void in my head. The noise which had dominated my thoughts was gone and it was often replaced by memories, many of them uncomfortable. Like fans looking for an autograph, memories of my childhood pressed into all the new silences in my brain. But gradually, I did start to read again. Gradually, I played the guitar. Gradually, I knew I was free. Whatever my father had done to me, it was all over for now.

When I returned to work there were a lot of cases waiting and by the time Jonathan Bowyer's trial came around, I was working long hours again and thought I was match fit.

At the Old Bailey, I met Mr Keenan, the prosecution barrister. We grabbed a takeaway coffee and then headed straight to chambers. We were at the heart of the capital's most ancient seat of justice. Here the walls were panelled, the armchairs were of worn leather. The only indication that this was the twenty-first century was a laptop in the corner. An assistant sat tapping at its keyboard.

We made ourselves comfortable, Mr Keenan propping his feet on a nearby stool.

'Newsflash,' he said gravely. 'The judge isn't allowing any mention of previous strangling.'

I stared at him in disbelief. My emotions felt so uncomplicated these days. Once, I would have experienced astonishment with a lot of banging inside my head. Now, it was just pure astonishment.

'But . . . he's been charged six times for strangling women!'

'You might well be surprised. But the judge says it's not to be mentioned, not by me and not by you on the witness stand. There is absolutely nothing we can do about it.'

'But . . .'

'But nothing. The judge is of the opinion that the jury would be unduly prejudiced if they learned how Bowyer has strangled previous partners.'

'Well . . . isn't it okay to be prejudiced by the truth?'

Mr Keenan shrugged helplessly and explained that we could not now call Jonathan Bowyer's previous partners to give evidence in court. No, we were in a legal minefield; all we could do was tiptoe.

'You are absolutely sure you didn't find any evidence of mental ill-health which would support a plea of diminished responsibility?' asked Mr Keenan. It was the defence psychiatrist's job to prove that Jonathan's mental health diminished his responsibility for the crime and therefore that he was guilty only of manslaughter. It was the prosecution's job to prove murder and this depended on my opinion that there was no mental disorder.

'Nothing at all.'

'Have you read the defence psychiatrist's report?'

There were plenty of experts, like Ari, who could be relied upon to find an obscure personality disorder in almost anyone: we are all very complex so that is not so hard. Jonathan Bowyer's defence psychiatrist had diagnosed one that was far from obscure: an emotionally unstable personality disorder, otherwise known as a borderline personality disorder. His report said that Mrs Bowyer had provoked Jonathan. Under such provocation, his personality disorder had diminished his ability to make decisions. Decisions like whether or not to kill her.

I really did not agree with this: I had already seen too many murderers blame their victims. I had found in Jonathan no evidence of any personality disorder, aside from being anti-social. He seemed to me to be a fully functioning, articulate and socially adept member of society. Although possibly a psychopath.

'What about the girl?' I asked. 'The deceased's daughter?'

'Jessica? She won't be called. She was questioned but couldn't say much more than the neighbours. She heard screaming and banging from their room, that's all. And frankly, she's been through enough.'

'Does she have support?' I asked.

'Well, that's not our focus . . .' Mr Keenan was thumbing through the bundle now.

'I can't help feeling concerned about her. Where is she?'

He looked up.

'With a foster family, I think. They put her in an emergency placement that night. Did I hear that she's moving in with a relative, something like that?'

He glanced vaguely in the direction of his assistant before returning to his paperwork.

The keyboard was suddenly silent.

'With an aunt,' the assistant said. 'She lives abroad but has come back to be with Jessica.'

The tapping resumed. It had hardly paused.

'Not our concern, Duncan,' Mr Keenan said absently, his nose in the bundle.

I raised my voice, very slightly.

'I'd like to see her,' I said. 'I feel I should, if only once. I won't retraumatize her, I just want to check things out and mobilize local services.'

Mr Keenan sighed and the sigh said: no.

I persisted. 'It really is important.'

'I'll set it up,' he muttered in a tone of great resignation, scribbling a note.

The mood in the room had become, if not tense, then irritable. It wasn't easy to insist on seeing Jessica but I knew I must try. It wasn't that I, personally, wanted to treat her: I was simply a doctor and a human being who wanted to reassure himself that a traumatized child had been given enough support and that the services which were designed to help really were rallying around her.

'Do you know the defence psychiatrist? Is he a name in your world?' asked Mr Keenan.

I shook my head. 'Never heard of him. I think he's from another part of the country.'

'The entire case,' said Mr Keenan, 'relies on Dr Sleet convincing the jury that Bowyer has a personality disorder.'

'And on me disproving it,' I added. I didn't think that would be too much of a problem.

14

The defence barrister glanced at the jury, as though checking all the class was paying attention, put her hands on her hips, turned to me, glaring, and then stood very still with raised eyebrows. I could remember teachers standing that way in class. Usually just before they delivered a detention.

Jury members leaned forward in anticipation.

'Are you really telling the court, Dr Harding, that the defendant *killed* his wife, *then* wrapped her in plastic, *then* dragged her into the bathroom, *then* rushed off to Portugal before his arrest several weeks later, are you really telling the court that he was *not* mentally ill? That this behaviour was *normal*? Is that what you are telling us?'

Her eyes were opened wide, her mouth gaped a little. She was a picture of incredulity.

I thought for a moment. Knowing that every word I said would be noted, possibly read back, perhaps used against me.

'I don't believe . . .' I began. Nope. Too hesitant. I glanced around the courtroom. Ari was sitting in the public gallery. He caught my eye and winked disarmingly. I tried to strengthen my voice. '. . . that I used the word "normal". But in my view, the defendant does not present with any mental disorder. And I could find no evidence that he suffered from a mental disorder at the time of the killing.'

'No evidence!' cried the defence barrister, eyebrows disappearing under her wig. '*No evidence!*'

Now she threw a quick, conspiratorial look of exasperation towards the jury.

'Did you not hear the evidence I have read to the court, Dr Harding? Dragging the body around, wrapping it up, rushing to Portugal – that seems perfectly clear evidence and I struggle to see why you cannot understand it.'

Very good. Straight out of RADA. And she had presented a defence line that I knew well – Ari used it all the time – and which was very hard to counter. The crime was so extraordinary that it could *only* be the act of a madman. Therefore, the defendant could not be held fully responsible for his actions.

This classic line plays well to jurors who may be influenced by the neat endings and clear motives of crime fiction. Faced with the muddles, the contradictions, the baffling nuances of real crime, which often appears to be without the focus of a well-defined motive, they agree with the defence. He must have been mad, or he wouldn't have done it. Would he?

I stood on the witness stand knowing that there would be years of wrestling with this one ahead of me and wondering if I really wanted to find myself in this position repeatedly. The position of someone who was trying to prove the non-existence of something, in this case, a personality disorder. As I faltered and reddened on the stand, I understood one of the reasons that Ari only took defence cases.

My hands felt clammy. I feared my face was glowing with sweat. I was experiencing the unpleasant feeling of my authority trickling away. Once more, Ari winked at me kindly.

'In my opinion,' I said, 'the defendant does not present with any mental disorder.'

All I could do now was repeat this phrase again and again. I did not know how to play any other game. If I had been more experienced, I might have reminded the court that Jonathan had managed to pack a suitcase, remember his passport, catch a train to the airport, buy a ticket, deal with airline staff, get to the required gate, catch his flight . . . I might have pointed to the clear decision-making and thought processes this required. And contrasted it with the defence's presentation of a man suffering from a mental illness which prevented him from making rational decisions.

But this was my first big case. I was intimidated by the size, gravity and antiquity of Court 1 at the Old Bailey. By the heaving public gallery, by the huge silence in the room when the barrister paused, by the press taking notes every time I opened my mouth. And by the defence barrister. Who was making me look inept.

She threw several statements at me which felt like accusations and sounded like questions and all I could do was repeat the same phrase: In my opinion . . . in my opinion . . . in my opinion . . .

Realizing that she had entirely shredded my authority and perhaps fearing that continuing in the same vein might have seemed bullying and cost her the jury's sympathy, the defence barrister told the judge that she had no further questions.

I could not look at Mr Keenan. I had let him down. I

had let Jessica's dead mother down. I had let Jessica down. I had allowed the defence barrister to beat me up like the kids on the housing estates where I was brought up. I had submitted then and I had submitted now. I had not stood my ground or shown the jury the truth I believed in. I had failed to advance the case against Jonathan at all.

Mr Keenan stood up for his re-examination and asked me gentle questions to redeem the situation, but I knew that the defence barrister's imprint on the jury was indelible. I hoped that Mr Keenan would dispose of the defence psychiatrist, Dr Sleet, in a similar manner. But first he was being questioned by his own side.

Dr Sleet was a small, slight man with a bow tie and a goatee beard. He was a caricature of the public's idea of a psychiatrist. Surely no one would listen to him.

I sat with the prosecution team and watched as, coaxed by the skilful barrister, he told the court about Jonathan's personality disorder. Under oath, he explained to the jury that the defendant had simply not been able to control himself at the time of the homicide – his ability to make a rational decision had been entirely compromised by his mental health. His wife's incessant nagging had provoked him to an extreme reaction, and his emotionally unstable personality disorder meant he was unable to consider the consequences of this reaction as the rest of us might. He agreed wholeheartedly when the barrister said that therefore the charge should surely be manslaughter. Yes, Dr Sleet stated, Mrs Bowyer had been a tragic victim not of Mr Bowyer but of the mental illness that controlled him.

When questioned by Mr Keenan, he answered succinctly, sticking to his opinion and not admitting to any other possibilities. His was not the performance of a heavyweight. But I knew he had been more convincing than me.

That was not the end of the case.

A defendant in a homicide trial won't always give evidence to the court: they might do themselves no favours in the witness box. But the defence had evidently enjoyed Jonathan's company as much as I had, and they wanted to share this with the jury.

There was a deep silence in the room as Jonathan took the stand, members of the jury watching him hawkishly. I was remembering something he had said to me: 'It's all about fucking diplomacy, see. I should work for the fucking Foreign Office.'

Within minutes he was charming the jury. I could see their fascination as his huge, expressive face and rollicking delivery took them on a joy ride of emotions.

He was humorous as he described meeting and marrying his wife, then he was suffering as the hard-working but henpecked husband who tried to meet her demands, next he was sad because the marriage that had started so well was going wrong despite his attempts to save it, next he was heroic as he tried to overlook his wife's 'yapping'. Then he was baffled because he had no memory of the night she died and finally he was broken-hearted at her death. Another RADA performance. If this had gone on for one more day, London theatre audiences would have been queuing outside the Old Bailey for the hottest ticket in town.

The defence finished and the court took a break. When we returned, Mr Keenan stood to cross-examine Jonathan and he had so much presence that I felt the whole room, including the jury, sit a little straighter. Jonathan had made everyone like him and now they guessed that Mr Keenan was setting out to undermine him.

Mr Keenan was relaxed and friendly at first, as though Jonathan had succeeded in charming him, too. There was an easy exchange. I thought of the way a cat plays with a mouse, letting it run backwards and forwards between its paws. Before killing it.

Slowly, cunningly, by asking repeated questions leading to the night of the homicide, all of which were offered in a reasonable, friendly tone, he was annoying Jonathan. And then making him angry. And then ramping up that anger. The defendant's voice was getting louder and his huge hands were grasping the edge of the witness box. I could see a white line across his knuckles. His answers became more waspish. Just as he had created a warmth in the courtroom when his own barrister had questioned him, now he was creating a different atmosphere. It reminded me of the tension in our house when my father rumbled around roaring dangerously, prior to punching me.

Mr Keenan asked about the crime itself.

'I fully understand from your evidence that you don't remember anything and I understand that it must be very annoying to be asked about an event you do not remember. But I hope you can see that it is my duty to the court to establish exactly when this memory loss occurred. I very much hope you can help me to pinpoint that moment?'

Jonathan glared at him, his eyes bulging.

'The evidence is incontrovertible that you placed your

hands around the deceased's throat and squeezed. That is so, isn't it?'

Jonathan continued to glare.

'That is so, isn't it?' repeated Mr Keenan politely.

'No comment,' breathed Jonathan. He sounded dangerous.

'Very well. Perhaps you can tell me if you remember raising your hands to Mrs Bowyer's throat?'

'No.'

'Placing them around her neck?'

'No.'

'And squeezing? You can't remember that either?'

'No.'

'Because you did squeeze. You squeezed and you squeezed; in fact, your hands tightened around your wife's neck until she could only gasp for breath. But you did not release her then. No, you continued to squeeze. Until there was no breath at all. You had squeezed the life out of her. Mrs Bowyer was dead and she couldn't "yap" any longer. Afterwards, you were left holding her lifeless body by the neck. I think most of us would remember that, Mr Bowyer.'

Mr Keenan had grown huge. He had become inflated by anger, by his belief in justice, by his fury that Mrs Bowyer had been killed. His voice was loud and he banged his fist hard on the desk.

'Mr Bowyer, you say you don't remember. But in your hands was a dead woman and you had strangled her! That's right, isn't it?'

'No comment.'

'And what then? When you saw what you had done? Did you dial 999 for an ambulance? Attempt resuscitation?

Yell for help, call the police, bang on the neighbours' doors, make some attempt to save the woman you had just strangled? No, you did not! Instead, you wrapped her in black plastic, dragged her to the bathroom, dumped her and left the property! That's right, isn't it?'

Jonathan's face was no longer still. The muscles in his jaw were working systematically, as if he were chewing on something gristly. His skin was red.

'No comment.'

'You had killed your wife and now, like a true coward, you ran away. You were on the run. On the lam and off to Portugal! Keen to escape the consequences. But instead you were arrested, cowering in a bed and breakfast, keeping your head down in the hope that it would all blow over. Despite your great cowardice, despite your attempts to hide yourself from justice, it didn't blow over! Did it?'

There was a pause as Jonathan chewed harder and turned redder. This lasted for perhaps fifteen seconds. And then he exploded. With a roar, he scrambled over the witness box, lunging at Mr Keenan. He was screaming so loudly that his voice echoed around the courtroom.

'I'll do you, you fucking bastard, I'll get that fucking wig off you and I'll tear it to pieces and I'll tear you with it, I'll fucking do you . . .'

I admired the composure of Mr Keenan. The rest of his team, and I was one of them, felt greatly inclined to exit rapidly, but he remained standing, motionless, watching Jonathan, saying nothing as at least four people attempted to restrain the defendant. Half-awake police officers came to life, court officials were startled into action and a couple of jury members looked ready to join in the affray. There was a moment when I thought Jonathan could overpower them all and really assault Mr Keenan before he was grounded and handcuffed.

Mr Keenan's face did not change as he was treated to a list of expletives, at least some of which were probably new to the jury and certainly to the judge. The jury was far enough away to experience no fear. They were simply enthralled by the drama.

You might think that Jonathan had just sworn his way to a very unfavourable verdict. However, the brilliant defence barrister was able to turn this outburst to her advantage.

'Ladies and gentlemen of the jury, you have witnessed here, in action, an emotionally unstable personality disorder. This, as our expert Dr Sleet has confirmed, is recognized as a very serious mental health condition. My client, Mr Bowyer, was intent on attacking my learned friend and, had he not been restrained by our most able officers . . .' (here she threw significant glances at the police officers, who were already starting to look sleepy again in the warm courtroom and now rapidly straightened) '. . . he would very unfortunately have succeeded, I do believe, in killing my learned friend!'

There was another significant glance, this time at Mr Keenan, which did not convince me that she thought Mr Keenan's escape unfortunate at all. Mr Keenan simply looked at her coldly and raised his eyebrows.

'And now, I suggest, the defendant has no memory of what has just occurred. What you have witnessed here in this room was exactly what happened on the night Mrs Bowyer died. Mr Bowyer is the unfortunate victim of a serious mental health problem. His inability to restrain himself, witnessed here by us all, has resulted in the death of a beloved wife and the great suffering which regret brings. He should be regarded with compassion and his condition treated . . .' And so on.

Despite Mr Keenan's Oscar-worthy performance, the defence outshone him. Jonathan Bowyer was found not guilty of murder, but guilty of manslaughter with diminished responsibility. His sentence was short. Logic dictates that anyone found guilty of that charge should go to hospital but I doubt Jonathan did. Or only for a brief assessment where he would probably have been found well enough to transfer to jail. He might only be kept there for a handful of years, undertaking none of the rehabilitation courses designed for those who intend to kill. Because he was not gulity of murder. For all I know, he could be out by now and have strangled an eighth woman.

15

'Don't be downcast. You've gained a lot of good experience from Jonathan Bowyer's case,' Ari told me. 'It's been very important for your learning curve.'

'If I'd been more confident and held my ground better then he might have been convicted of murder. Emotionally unstable personality disorder? Jonathan's a dangerous psychopath and he's going to be back out there soon and it feels like my fault.'

Ari shook his head.

'Maybe he'll be assessed as unsafe for release and kept inside. Listen, Duncan, you did your best and that's all any of us can do. Now, follow the golden rule: don't take it home with you.'

I tried to follow the golden rule but knew I had to meet Jessica before I could stop worrying about the case.

I had already determined that I would not cause her the anguish of asking her about the night her mother died. I had tried to see events from her point of view, though. The argument, her mother's screams, the abrupt, awful silence. Peeling back the plastic to see her mother's purple face, huge finger marks on the neck. Did she fear Jonathan's return? Did she crouch by the body, hopelessly waiting for a response? Sirens. Her removal from the scene. Arrival at a stranger's house. A new bedroom, a new bed. No mother.

How could Jessica ever recover from this? How could I help her?

She was tiny and birdlike. Her eyes were dark and her facial expression strangely hollow, even horrified, as though the homicide had only happened last night. She sat very still and barely looked at me. Her answers to my gentle questions were short, half whispered. She was more mouse than girl.

I was sure that she did need specialist support. I found that she had not been signed up with a GP in her new area. The Child and Adolescent Mental Health Service knew nothing of her either. I was glad that at least I could set help in motion for her: this would give her a hope of overcoming her trauma or anyway learning to co-exist with it. Maybe, just maybe, she could grow towards a fulfilling life.

As for Jonathan, I really felt he was beyond any help. I reached a new state of hopelessness. *Pace*, Alice, but I believed now that no amount of talking, training or intervention would change Jonathan, or many like him. Which led me to a burning question. And on this my future rested. If I had met Jonathan when he was still a child, would it have been possible to work with him to prevent him becoming an adult psychopath?

'Maybe,' said John Brontë. 'We still haven't discovered a way to treat adult psychopathy, of course, but diverting a child away from psychopathy before it becomes an untreatable adult condition must be one of the highest achievements of child psychiatry.'

It was summer and we were in the garden. Thankfully, John had not poured me a whisky, but a glass of cold mineral water. We were watching his new bird table as we talked: it was positioned a few feet from a hedge and tiny birds flitted from hedge to table and back constantly.

John had recently been beaten up by a patient, a seventeen-year-old who had hidden a knife and sprung at him without warning. He had been attacked before but this time his confidence, as well as his physical health, had been significantly affected.

'I want to work, I love my work, but how can I do it if I feel fear?' he asked. 'Oh, the knife wound has healed, my broken elbow has healed, although my arm may never be quite the same.' His attacker had thrown him across the table and stood on the arm John had used to defend himself. 'But fear . . . that's not so easy to manage.'

This incident did not make me reconsider my work in forensic medicine although I knew attack was an occupational hazard. A consultancy in forensic psychiatry was within sight now, I was just a year or so away from it. But John's experience made me determined to be more careful. I told John that we should always insist on having panic buttons in consulting rooms – as well as the certainty that pressing them would bring help.

'Yes,' he agreed. His tone was benign but without hope. 'We should not change career. We should insist on panic buttons.'

He looked much older. That robust, razor-sharp edge of his was missing. Perhaps because of the attack, but perhaps because he had taken a sabbatical from work. His new hobby was identifying visitors to his bird table. I understood his fears but this change irritated me. John was a brilliant psychiatrist, he should be working with children, not looking at beaks and feathers all day.

'Tell me about the interventions which help children to change,' I persisted. 'Because in adult psychiatry I'm seeing some offenders who can't, won't change.'

'Are you losing your sense of therapeutic hope, Duncan?'

'A little.'

'Well, let me reassure you that there are plenty of therapeutic interventions for children and they are developing all the time but, for me, the underlying question is: would this young offender benefit from some tight boundaries? Even, yes, lock and key? Therapy works best when a child feels safe. When they've been out on the wild streets, when home is chaotic, some tight boundaries can feel very good and safe and that is what a child needs before you can begin to help them.'

I was startled.

'You mean prison?'

'Maybe. There are children's secure units that do such good work. People get upset at the very idea, but security is the bedrock of therapeutic work.'

'And how successful is that therapeutic work?'

'Well, it's a lot more likely to be successful with children than adults.'

So, working with children really was about hope and about change.

'John, you did once say, when I first met you, that I should consider child psychiatry. I didn't agree with you at all . . .' Oh, how I had resisted the idea. '. . . but now I see you were right.'

'Really?' He ran a hand through his thick white hair. 'That is good to hear, not least because I'm so often wrong these days. But are you telling me that . . . ?'

'When I've finished my training in adult forensic psychiatry, I want to specialize in children and adolescents.'

His face broke into a huge smile. 'Forensically?'

My voice was firm. 'Yes. I want to be a forensic psychiatrist for children.'

'Oh, I'm very glad you've decided this. What changed your mind?'

'My dad hit me so hard in the head that years later I needed brain surgery. As I lay in my hospital bed I was wondering why no one picked up my distress signals when I was a kid. There were so many obvious signs that something was wrong at home. I wouldn't use the school toilets, not ever. I pretended to be sick every Monday so that I wouldn't have to take my clothes off for PE. I was certainly a kid waving a red flag and no one noticed or cared. That's why I want to be someone who listens to children.'

He nodded.

'Then something else happened. The psychopath I was telling you about. Jonathan. When he murdered his wife, her eight-year-old daughter, Jessica, was in the house. She was found clinging to her mother's body. I felt so concerned about her that I insisted on seeing her after the trial. I know it will be hard for her to get through this trauma but . . . well, she's young and there is hope. If she gets the right help. On the other hand, Jonathan's unlikely to change, no matter what help he has. That made me feel that therapeutic hope lies with children.'

'Good, good, we must all practise with therapeutic hope. Although I am sure you understand that, even with support, Jessica's road will be a hard one.'

‘I made CAMHS and her GP aware of her.’

‘But how will she fit in at school, I wonder? Because the other children will soon know that there’s something different about Jessica. They’ll guess she’s vulnerable, detached, a bit of an outsider, they may even sense that she has experienced trauma. And will that mean they are kind to her? Sadly not. The school, her carer, everyone will have to be very alert to cruelty and bullying.’

‘So the other children will detect she’s been traumatized and they’ll try to make things worse?’

‘There is no disputing child’s inhumanity to child. You remember that.’

Yes, I remembered that.

‘Do you think I should contact the –?’

‘Stop! You’ve done enough! Some would say too much: as the prosecution’s psychiatrist, you have no business addressing the victim’s problems.’

A flapping of wings and a huge pigeon which had been threatening to land on the bird table from a low branch disappeared.

‘He’ll return, I’m afraid,’ said John. ‘To steal from the song birds. Brutes are part of life’s ceaseless rhythm. Although of course, he doesn’t know he’s a thief: he’s just hungry.’

I smiled broadly.

‘That’s exactly what my grandfather would have said.’

Grandad had been quick to love and slow to condemn. My rock. His little house, built for men returning from the war and intended only as temporary accommodation, had lasted him a lifetime. At night he worked repairing the railway; in the day he took good care of his house, and good care of me too. The place was small and so thin-walled it was almost made of paper, but it had been a fortress for me, a sanctuary from the violence. And now, here I was with John in his sanctuary. I glanced at him anxiously as he poured us more water. Did I detect a shaking hand? The thought alarmed me. John wasn't allowed to get old and die the way Grandad had.

He said: 'Oh, but I am so pleased at your big decision. I believe it is the right one.'

This felt like a significant day, a significant moment. We watched the tiny birds as they squeaked and chattered noisily in their own language. Now I had stated my decision out loud, I knew that I was going to do it. I was going to qualify as a forensic psychiatrist for adults . . . and then become a forensic psychiatrist for children.

I met with the training director and learned that there were two routes to my new goal. One was shorter than the other. When I became a consultant in forensic psychiatry, I could just do two extra years of training with children and young people to practise forensically with them. The longer route would mean I continued forensic work with adults while undertaking a full higher training in child and adolescent psychiatry. Once I had attained that, I could specialize in forensic work with young people.

The long route meant that I would be able to work with children, adolescents or adults in forensic psychiatry. I would have cradle to grave training, be able to unpick the mind across a person's lifetime. I would be on the GMC specialist register as a child and adolescent expert, and as a forensic expert.

I chose the long route.

'You're a glutton for punishment!' cried Ari Good. He had been unable to hide his surprise at my decision.

'Of course, I'll continue to work with you on adult forensic work while I train with children,' I assured him.

He squinted back at me. 'Well, it's going to be very hard. I really don't know why you would choose it.' He was shaking his head. 'It's going to cost you years!'

I laughed.

'Your life will be a series of six-month placements – like a young doctor. But you're not young! They'll have you in outpatients, inpatients, acute hospital settings . . . then there's all the specialist clinics. Obsessive-compulsive disorder, ADHD, autistic spectrum disorder, you name it, you'll go there. And that's before you even start to work forensically. You'll be pulled from pillar to post until you're dizzy. Reconsider, Duncan! I beg, you, reconsider!'

But I did not reconsider. I knew this was a journey worth taking. Because it would be full of fascinating cases.

16

In medicine, working and training are essentially the same thing. I was in the early stages of both working with and training for child patients when Jack came along.

'Same shirt again, Doctor!' said Jack's dad jovially as he entered the consulting room. This was pitched as a joke but by now I had learned that Michael's jokes were usually poorly disguised jibes. I smiled and said nothing, while silently promising myself that I would certainly go shopping for shirts. And even buy different colours, to make the difference obvious.

Jack had entered leaning on his mother's arm and was finding his seat. He was feeling the chair before he sat in it, tapping his white stick on the floor around it, checking its height and angle before he sat down.

His mother, Angela, said: 'We're a bit late again, sorry, Doctor. I'm sure you have much better things you could be doing with your time. But he had to have a cigarette before he came in.'

She glanced at her husband, who avoided her eye. He sat down and I inhaled that familiar smell of my childhood: smoke and the sweetness of nicotine.

Angela and Michael were very smartly dressed. He wore an immaculate suit, the immaculate suit of a chauffeur. Angela wore a tailored dress and her perfume always entered the room before she did. She worked in the cosmetics hall of an Oxford Street department store, a place I had sometimes, on passing through, marvelled at for its pristine white light, competing scents and perfectly coiffed women. And now, here was one of those women in my office, looking just as she did in the store: pristine, coiffed and smelling expensive.

Michael had started life as possibly London's best-dressed taxi driver – or maybe the suits had come later. He had spotted a gap in the market and set up his own business, sending out limousines and their drivers to pick up VIPs and celebrities. Now he had a thriving business. The family occasionally arrived in one of the long, gleaming limousines: I knew that because it caused a small sensation among the reception staff, who were disappointed when Adele did not step out of it.

'If I like the look of a celeb then I do the job myself,' Michael had explained at an early session, reeling off the famous names he had driven around London. 'Otherwise, the boys do the driving and I sit there in the office wishing I was out on the road. That's what happens when you get big. There isn't time to do the job you love any more.'

Life had changed dramatically for the Porter family about two years ago. First, Jack's younger brother, Nathan, had been diagnosed with leukaemia. He was five. Then, just when Nathan was coming out of hospital after intensive treatment and the Porters were allowing themselves to hope all would be well, something had happened to Jack. Initially it had seemed like a small incident. The boy, then aged nine, had simply been poked in the eye with a paintbrush during a school art class. The eye was red and swollen, nothing more, but, as the swelling went down, he complained that he could not see.

He had been subjected to a battery of tests by ophthalmologists. But the reason for his sight loss was a mystery. There was nothing wrong with the cornea, no evidence of a tumour, no damage to the retina and no enduring signs of trauma anywhere. Every test result seemed to say that Jack could see. But he insisted he couldn't.

His blindness was therefore described as 'non-organic'. And, not so long ago, it would have been called 'hysterical'. In other words, there was no physical reason for it and so it was considered possible that Jack had, consciously or unconsciously, chosen to be blind. And there was another, even less palatable possibility. Was he simply pretending?

Jack was a candidate for some therapeutic work with the psychology department at the hospital but they had declined him as a patient. The conflicting explanations and possibilities – organic condition or psychological disturbance? – meant that Jack's parents, who could not shake off the idea that we had missed some physical cause for the blindness, would only be happy if a doctor saw him. There was no established pathway for such a case and the psychologists were pleased to pass Jack to a keen child psychiatrist.

Michael and Angela were plagued by the question: was this blindness real or not? Their emotional reactions to it varied. Naturally, they were worried; at other times they were hurt, baffled, angry or frustrated. For the last eighteen months they had, however, chosen to believe their son. This belief sometimes wavered but they seemed to accept that Jack's world was now so blurred that he needed a white stick. Recently he had stopped attending school altogether and his mother had begun studying at home with him.

Angela had certainly convinced herself that Jack's blindness had a physical cause. She often said: 'Look, Duncan, don't you think it would be better if we worked with a doctor qualified in sight impairment?'

And in the very first session she had turned to her son reassuringly and said: 'It's not that we think you're making anything up, Jack. But seeing Duncan is a sort of screening process. We have to get through this before they'll take a closer look at your eyes.'

Jack was helping me understand how different child psychiatry was from adult psychiatry. He was illustrating the fact that there is seldom any point assessing a child in isolation. You can try. But sooner or later, it usually becomes essential to work within the context of the child's family unit, and perhaps their school and friendship units too.

When it comes to treatment, the same applies: you work with the whole family. And treatment, for children, tends to be less about medication and more about psychology. And so I saw the Porter family weekly for many months.

Younger brother Nathan had pulled through his leukaemia and, although he was of course carefully watched for its return, life was back to normal for him. He attended just a few of our sessions. And his presence transformed them. The door would bang open and Nathan was first to burst in, wearing full football kit, often mud on his knees, his mother never far behind him, tutting and trying to wipe it off with a tissue. He was lively to the point of effervescence.

'How was the game?' I'd ask, and that was all it took; he was immediately off, describing the match in enthusiastic detail, often jumping up to demonstrate the best kicks. We watched him, enthralled: he was not showing off; he was genuinely keen for us to share the pleasure he took in football. It was impossible not to laugh and sigh with him.

Unselfconsciously, unintentionally, Nathan stole all the oxygen whenever he was in the room. While Jack sat very still, speaking little. Jack was large and rather lumbering, not, he had explained, good at sport like his nimble younger brother. He wore baggy clothes of indeterminate colours. As if he was trying to be as dull as possible.

I thought it might not be a coincidence that Jack's blindness had first occurred just as the family was pulling out of an acute medical crisis. The amount of attention lively Nathan garnered must also be relevant. It seemed to me that Jack had created his own blindness because he needed it. Blindness changed the dynamic in the family. And it enabled him to withdraw. I observed this, but I did not know the reason for any of it.

He often sat silently at our sessions, saying nothing even when invited to speak. Today the family was late, Angela blaming Michael's need for a cigarette, and an antagonistic dialogue had ensued between the parents, as it so often did. I noticed how, throughout this, Jack looked ahead unseeingly, as if lack of sight robbed him of hearing or the need to participate.

'You did a survey back at school, didn't you, Jack-o?' said his mother. 'Wasn't it about how many children had parents who smoked?'

She was looking at Jack, but Angela's real target was Michael. It was easy to see how she was using her ten-year-old son as a conduit for the anger intended for her husband.

'Oh yeah, and you're going to tell me that I was the only bloody smoker in the survey, right?' demanded Michael.

Jack leaned forward as if the chair was planning to rock and unseat him. He remained silent.

'Just one other dad smoked, I think?' his mother prompted.

Finally, Jack spoke. 'Eight parents smoked.' His voice was low. It lacked energy, as if the subject was without interest.

I thought we might as well follow this line, since the family had begun it.

'How do you feel about your dad smoking, Jack?' I asked.

He said nothing. He wound the hem of his sweatshirt around his hand, frowning a little. Jack seldom, if ever, smiled.

I waited for him to reply, but Angela was impatient.

'It does worry you, really,' she informed Jack. 'You know how it's not good for Dad's health. Luckily he always goes outside for a cigarette, so we don't have to inhale a lungful of toxins too.'

I said: 'Thanks, Angela, but let's hear what Jack has to say about Dad's cigarettes.'

Jack looked straight ahead, not focusing, not seeing. Or pretending he could not do these things.

The silence in the consulting room went on a long time, as silences with the Porter family often did. Angela found this particularly hard.

'I don't know what you normally do, Doctor,' she said at last. 'But sitting here doing nothing seems like a complete waste of taxpayers' money.'

I said: 'I'm giving Jack time to think before he answers. Some people need that space.'

We waited. Jack looked at the ground, Michael looked at the ceiling and Angela looked around the room, her jaw set.

Finally, she could bear it no longer. 'Oh, for God's sake, hurry up and answer, Jack.'

Jack said nothing. Neither did I. Angela's face became really miserable as the silence continued, but the next outburst came from Michael.

'Can't you just open your bloody eyes!' he snapped.

Jack blinked and slumped back in his chair as if he had been hit. His eyes had been open all along, of course.

'He can't see!' exclaimed Angela in exasperation.

Whenever I asked Jack questions, I created the space for him to answer them. From what I had seen of the family dynamic, I thought it was important for him to know that he had a place and a voice, and that his voice would still be heard even without the loudhailer of physical disability.

'Christ. Just calm down,' said Michael to his wife now.

I had been fooled into thinking Angela was calm when we first started working together. She had seemed unruffled. She wore a lot of perfectly applied make-up and, whatever happened, her mask was unchanging. Gradually, I learned more about her. When her father had died very suddenly during her childhood, she told me she had developed a sort of emotional detachment. And, years later, she seemed to be dealing with Nathan's leukaemia and now Jack's eyes with the same detachment. It helped her retain control – of herself, of others. Lots of people, after a trauma, try to exercise control: they don't want to feel helpless in the face of trauma again. But it seemed to me that Angela's attempts to maintain control of the family were one source of anger between the couple. And there was a lot of anger.

'For God's sake, relax,' Michael told his wife. 'I couldn't get uptight like you. Do that when you're driving and clients won't come back. Plus everyone knows that's when accidents happen.'

'We're not driving! We're not going anywhere!' Angela hissed, her voice low and taut.

'Calm down!' insisted her husband again. He glanced at me and then back at his wife.

'Duncan calls himself a doctor, so I'm guessing he must be. Although I daresay I'd done the Knowledge long before he went to medical school.'

I doubted that. Michael can't have been more than a few years older than me.

Now Angela reorganized herself in her seat and recomposed her features into the calm expression that I knew was not really calm.

'Jack, I'd be interested to hear how you feel about Dad smoking,' I said. I was determined to keep the space open for him. 'Your mum's made her feelings clear, now it's your turn to speak.'

Silence. Forever. And then, just when his parents' faces were pictures of despair, he said: 'Well . . . sometimes I don't like the smell because –'

Angela jumped in.

'The smell's dreadful and it gets everywhere. But I notice he manages not to smoke when he's got Simon Cowell in the back seat!'

Her anger had been lurking, ready to ambush us, and now it had effectively stopped Jack from speaking. Yet again.

'Angela, please could you wait, because Jack was just saying something . . .' I held up a hand to halt her. We all turned to Jack.

Silence.

'What were you going to say about the smell of my cigarettes?' prompted his father eventually.

But it seemed Jack had nothing more to say. Michael felt the cigarette packet in his pocket. Angela looked ostentatiously at the clock. And I sat wondering yet again what role Jack's blindness played in the family. Why he may have found it necessary – entirely unconsciously, I was sure – to be ill just as his brother was getting better.

I didn't want to place Jack in a spotlight now – he would never have been comfortable with that – but his parents had to stop filling Jack's space with their own battles.

Gradually, I learned that, before Nathan was diagnosed with leukaemia, the family home had become a battle ground. The parents had argued. A lot. Over everything. Over who would pick up the children, over Michael's Sunday mornings with his driver mates, over Angela's expenditure on clothes, over how many hours she should work and how many hours he spent in the office . . . there seemed to be a battle for control of their lives.

I guessed that with the devastating news of Nathan's illness, all that had stopped. I knew only too well the terrible silence that can wrap itself around a life and death situation. All the quarrels, the chatter, the one-upmanship: when death threatens it brings a new perspective and, sometimes, silence. In the case of the Porters, I suspected the terrible silence had brought with it a truce, even a reconciliation, and consequently great relief to Jack. As Nathan began to recover, perhaps the rows had started again. Or perhaps Jack simply feared they would. Unconsciously, he had chosen his weapon. His blindness prolonged the parental worry that had bound them together and it enabled Jack to disengage from whatever painful events went on around him.

And so I spent many weeks ostensibly focusing on Jack but really working with Michael and Angela on their angry relationship. Jack sat quietly while his parents talked. This work with his parents was long and painfully slow, but I believe that it was both helpful and healing for Jack. Over the months, I saw their battles ease. Gradually, they were starting to come together again. And then something remarkable happened.

One day we were discussing how Jack's home schooling was going. Angela was telling me that Jack had wanted to know how the heart worked and they had bought a lamb's heart at the butcher's so that he could feel the chambers and ventricles. It had been entirely possible for him to understand the heart without actually seeing it. He explained this to us with something that, if not actually enthusiasm, might have been its poor relation. His parents were impressed at his interest. They exchanged glances and nodded approval. And Jack, although he could not see it, evidently sensed this.

I responded rapidly.

'Does it ever seem that your sight's a bit better or a bit worse?'

I expected nothing. So I was as surprised as his parents when he said: 'It might be getting a bit clearer.'

There was a shocked silence.

'Jack?' whispered his mother.

'I mean, just a bit,' he said carefully.

'Oh Jack-o!' Angela cried. 'I always believed that you –'

I waved an urgent hand to stop her. Please, Angela. Please, Michael. Give Jack some space and don't load your feelings on to him.

'What's actually clearer?' I asked.

'Everything.'

'What do you mean?'

Silence.

'You mean this room is clearer? I'm clearer? Outside is clearer? Or do you mean that you understand more now?'

He said nothing. It was all I could do to stop his excited parents replying for him. They both opened their mouths and I shot them a glance. Slowly, their mouths shut. And then Jack spoke again.

'It's blue. Outside, I mean. I can see the clouds behind you. Everything's still blurry, but I can see.'

There was another moment of disbelief and then the room was transformed. I realized that, when Michael smiled, he had a warm, pleasant face – he had mostly scowled through our sessions. Angela, for perhaps the first time, relaxed completely as she melted into tears. She leaned over and hugged her son. And there was another first. Jack smiled. A breakthrough. After months and months of anger and silence, the room had turned in an instant from monochrome into colour. The sky was blue!

I was confident that Jack was aware of the effect he'd had and that he took pleasure in it. As for me, I knew our sessions would not continue for much longer. Some barrier had been broken, some need had been nourished, some fear had been released.

There could be any number of theories about Jack's blindness and we'll never know the reason for sure. Training in psychiatry is training to live with uncertainty, often without resolution, and always with a sense of wonder at the human mind. I did think I had managed to shift the family's tectonic plates by providing a safe space for them to interact differently. I hoped that the work I did with Jack's parents had led to a greater sense of hope and positivity within the family unit. And Jack no longer felt that sickness in the family was the only way to manage his parents' anger.

I did not think there could be another case as strange as Jack's. But, soon afterwards, Emma came along.

17

Emma had started to have seizures about a year ago. Their intensity and frequency caused great distress to her family, friends and school, as well as to Emma herself. It was assumed that she must be epileptic. But physical seizures show spikes in brain activity: apparently, Emma had no such spikes. In fact, all the tests and evidence used to diagnose epilepsy were negative. The seizures were not physical. They were something else.

Were they caused by depression or anxiety? This would be very unusual, but if there were such an underlying cause then medication might help. I arranged to meet Emma with her family, take her history and talk to her. After which, I did not diagnose depression or anxiety.

So we were looking at solutions which did not involve medication. What could be causing these seizures? Was there some unconscious driver? Or was Emma just pretending? It was the same unpleasant question that I had faced with Jack.

Emma's family was completely different from Jack's. They were much easier to deal with. Her parents were seriously concerned about Emma but still gave her the space to think and to talk freely. And Emma was a much more talkative child than Jack.

The family lived in a housing association home and both parents were kind people who had worked hard all their lives. Emma's mother had been greatly upset by her twelve-year-old daughter's seizures and, like so many parents of disturbed adolescents, she cherished the fantasy that she could love and hug the problem away with compassion.

It didn't take me long to see that she was contributing to the problem, not alleviating it. I was learning a lot about children now and learning fast, and this was my learning curve with Emma. Her case demonstrated that the way those around a child react to problems can greatly affect outcomes, perhaps reinforcing the disturbance and prolonging it by years.

By now I was coming to the conclusion that, where a child has a mental health challenge, parents should not respond with displays of overt emotion. It is nearly always the case that adults need to moderate their response, whether that is anger and shouting or love and compassion. I am not suggesting they turn into robots. They may feel very deeply. But I was learning that it is usually best to filter some of that emotion so that it is not over-expressed to the child.

In Emma's case, her mother's knee-jerk love and compassion were unfiltered. When Emma had a seizure, her mother screamed, sobbed, held her hand and repeatedly wailed how much she loved her. Many mothers would feel that way. But by expressing these feelings so overtly, she was unconsciously giving the seizures an emotional charge and offering Emma the secondary gain that, by having seizures, she would receive a demonstration that she was passionately loved.

This led to the question: was Emma having seizures

because unconsciously she did not feel loved and cared for and she desperately needed this reassurance? As time went by, I became sure that this was not the case. She certainly had good enough parents – and that is all any of us can hope for.

At our initial sessions, Emma's quiet and steady father was ready to entertain the possibility that her seizures had some psychological cause, but Emma and, even more so her mother, was not. Her mother simply refused to accept that anything so physical, so shocking, so upsetting to the child, could be caused by the child herself.

The mother often burst into tears and grabbed Emma's hand during sessions: 'Ems, it's going to be all right, I promise you, darling, we're going to be strong and get through this together.' She dabbed at her eyes with an endless stream of tissues. 'I just want her to be okay, Doctor. Please!' Followed by more sobs.

I turned to Emma, who was dry-eyed.

'Can you describe what it's like to have a seizure?'

Although only twelve, going on thirteen, puberty was advanced and Emma looked more like fourteen or fifteen. She spoke with confidence.

'So, it's like, the world goes red, then black, and I don't see anything at all.'

'Does this happen just any time?'

'I never know when it's going to happen.'

'Do you think there might be something that can trigger the seizures?'

Emma's hair was carefully arranged to look careless and it fell across her face now. She sometimes fell into the pout used by so many teenagers on social media. But overall she was a relaxed, natural but somewhat troubled child. She shook her head.

'Nothing I can think of, they just come out of the blue.'

I talked to the mother and father about their own lives and did not uncover any traumas which might be expressed through the way they parented Emma. There was no explanation, except my firm belief that the great concern her mother felt was being over-expressed in a way that reinforced the behaviour.

I discussed this case with my supervisor.

'I'm baffled. They're a well-balanced, loving family. Whatever I look for, I find a blank. We're not getting anywhere.'

She smiled.

'That's just when we have to persevere. When we think we're not getting anywhere. Something will give, I promise. Get the mother to stop emoting all over the daughter; that could just be the change which triggers a breakthrough.'

She was right. Two things soon happened. First, Emma's mother began to accept that there might be a psychological, if entirely unconscious, reason for the seizures and that we were here to find that reason. Second, she really did start trying hard not to panic when Emma had a seizure. This was certainly helping to ease any strain between the parents – tension had developed because Emma's father had been concerned by his wife's reactions. But I would not say that the parental relationship was in any difficulty: a child's illness can so often reflect unhappiness between parents, but I did not feel that this was the root cause of the problem.

'Any change?' asked my supervisor after a few weeks.

'Well, I do notice that, as her mother relaxes and stops sobbing, Emma's beginning to relax too.'

'Good. She's starting to feel safe. Soon, she'll trust you enough to talk.'

I was still so new to child psychiatry that I had little faith. It was going to turn into another case like Jack: week after week after week when nothing happened. But, quite suddenly, Emma did start to talk.

I had noticed that the seizures had a slight tendency to happen on a Sunday night. I could not help suspecting that they were associated with some problem at school. We often discussed this possibility, but Emma always denied it.

Today we were talking about friends and social media as we had before, but now she asked, casually: 'Do you know what Snapchat is?'

I sensed at once that this was critical. But her casual tone was important and I would have to match it when I responded. So, I smiled. Yes, I knew about Snapchat.

'It's supposed to disappear right away, isn't it?'

That was what kids seemed to love about Snapchat. They could send pictures to each other and the images were there . . . and then they weren't. But by now I was sure. There was something critical in Emma's casual mention of Snapchat.

'Supposed to,' I agreed. 'But I think there might be ways of capturing the image, right?'

'Yeah.' She paused. 'I didn't know that. I didn't know it could be saved.'

I was sure this was significant. So were her parents. I was aware that they were suddenly sitting very still.

I asked, gently: 'Have you ever sent an image which someone saved?'

She nodded.

'Yeah. Yeah, I did once.'

'What was it?'

'A video.'

'What did that show, Emma?'

There was a pause. I hoped I hadn't lost her. She was staring down at her fingers and her face was reddening.

'It was me, naked.'

Suddenly Emma's mother seemed to inflate, like a cartoon character or a bouncy castle. I could feel her presence, bobbing at my side. Sense her starting to sob. I glanced at her and she opened her mouth to wail, as if she would burst if she did not. I held my hand out straight. Stop! And, surprisingly, she did.

'It's okay, Emma,' I said. 'You can tell us. Who did you send it to? Your mum and dad need to know.'

'A boy, just a boy in my class. I thought he liked me. But he sent it to a friend, and they sent it to someone else, then someone else and . . . and then these girls got it. They're a sort of group. A group of girls who all sit together and they're all pretty and a bit scary and everyone wants to impress them and . . . anyway, they got it. And then . . . then life was hell.'

So, there it was. Presented to us on a plate.

The parents disclosed this bullying to the school. The seizures did not stop right away, but slowly they eased. Finally, they stopped altogether. The video itself would never disappear but Emma's pent-up distress was gradually dissipating as she shared her feelings with her family and friends.

She was being badly bullied and if she had not (unconsciously) externalized her disturbance into very public and violent seizures, there would have been a great risk that the misery might have been internalized. It is usually detached and insular children who so tragically kill themselves as a result of bullying. Being brought up by good enough parents was one of the factors that helped Emma to choose the safer, external expression of her pain. For other children, there may be different factors and so even outstanding parenting cannot, of course, necessarily prevent suicide. But Emma's kind parents certainly helped her.

They were delighted and grateful that we had sorted out this problem. Of course, I felt good too. The treatment had simply involved developing a framework of understanding. And a good enough theory to help her good enough parents offer Emma a healthier and more moderated emotional support structure.

That was an interesting clinic to train in, but I seldom stayed anywhere longer than six months. My next stop was the Tourette's Syndrome clinic. Here my new boss was clever, competent . . . and cold.

'You'll enjoy working here,' he said, looking me up and down. It sounded like an instruction. Every word he spoke was delivered like an order, as if you were supposed to jump to attention. He wore a tweedy jacket and a tie with flying pheasants on it. He was one of the few consultants left who dressed as if they had just stopped at the hospital en route for the leather armchairs of their club.

I nodded obediently to show that I intended to enjoy working here.

'Bit older than most of my trainees,' he said, still observing me closely. I wondered what it was like to be his patient.

'I took a roundabout route,' I explained. 'I spent almost ten years in neurological research.'

He did not invite me to enlarge on this.

'You moved into child psychiatry because you want to help young patients. Well, here in the Tourette's Clinic, that's just what we do. You'll find it very satisfying.'

This was an instruction it proved easy to follow. I learned that Tourette's is a syndrome that can usually be managed and so it was possible to change lives for the better. And, under that consultant's watchful eye, I discovered even more about the importance of the family support structure and systemic thinking.

Tourette's can take many different forms – not everyone involuntarily yells out words or phrases. Ben had a complex motor tic.

'I can't help it, I can't help it!' he cried as he arched his whole body forwards and touched his forehead on to his right knee. He was ten and this happened several times a day. At home. Also at school. Where, as a result of this strange, repeated action, he had been so badly bullied that he was on the edge of depression. I was reluctant, and still am, to diagnose depression in children, but I am afraid Ben was very close indeed to that diagnosis.

His family and I devised a strategy for dealing with his tic. In the past they had laughed it off as a quirky mannerism, but as the tic got worse they had started to worry. Once they felt anxiety, Ben of course sensed that. They might have tried to tell him it was okay with a smile, but anxiety was never far from the surface.

I explored all this with them, listening and not judging, remaining neutral. I explained the impact that any kind of emotionally driven response would have, and how children can sniff out anxiety however well it is hidden. Anxiety – in fact, paying any kind of attention to the tic – would only reinforce it.

So they agreed not to respond to it at all. Not positively. Not negatively. When he started to arch his back, they would simply ignore the tic as though it didn't exist. They even signed a written contract with Ben. Yes, they really signed a piece of paper saying that they would take absolutely no notice. The solemnity and symbolism of this signing was important.

Result: the tics became less frequent.

'But,' said the consultant when I checked in with him, 'it still happens?'

'It still happens, especially at school, and that's where he suffers most.'

'Hmmm. You've worked with the family. I should concentrate on Ben alone now.'

I arranged to do some individual work with Ben.

'Do you get any warning at all, even a very small one, before it happens?' I asked. Some people have an aura which warns them of an epileptic seizure and the same can be true of complex motor tics.

'Yeah, just a moment before.'

'What's it like?'

'Sort of tingly . . . it feels really weird.'

'Where is the tingle?'

He pointed to the left side of his neck.

'Does it last for a second before the tic starts?'

He thought hard.

'Maybe two seconds.'

'Right, let's try to think of a voluntary movement – that's one you want to do and can control – for the very moment you feel the tingle. Before your head starts to duck towards your knee.'

He stared at me.

'It's a new movement which will be entirely within your control. It might just counteract the tic.'

After much discussion, he agreed to try to look up the moment he felt the tingle. To look up, holding his head and back straight.

At first, he reported that this was impossible. It didn't help at all. But he persevered. He was jubilant when he finally succeeded, just once, in using the technique to short-circuit the tic. As soon as he had experienced success, he was keen for more. Within a few weeks, he found he could usually control the tic at home. But not at school.

'How about keeping a diary?' I suggested. 'Write down exactly when you have the aura and the movements. And then give yourself a score for counteracting it. Ten is the top grade you can give.'

He said: 'I quite often get tens at home but I'm getting zeros at school.'

'Keep trying and remember to write it down in the diary.'

Ben became an investigator of his own illness. The Hawthorne effect is an interesting, disputed theory. According to this theory, being the subject of a study can alter the very behaviour that is being studied. It is called the Hawthorne effect because it first emerged many years ago as a result of productivity research at the Hawthorne Works, an electric company in Illinois. Output increased whenever the researchers studied the workers and it was concluded that output increased *because* researchers were studying the workers. The results of that experiment have been challenged but, whether it's a true theory or not, it seemed to work for Ben. He was the subject of his own study and his behaviour was gradually modified accordingly.

After about four months of weekly sessions, Ben's complex motor tic disappeared. Initially it was replaced by the counteracting movement, but in time, as people around him did not respond at all when he looked up and straightened his back, that movement, too, drifted away. So did the aura. It was as though the counteracting movement extinguished the flame of the complex motor tic.

When we ended the sessions, I explained to Ben and the family that it was possible, if not likely, that the tic might reappear in the future: the risk of this diminishes substantially after the age of twelve.

'He won't be back,' the experienced consultant assured me. 'If the tic recurs, the boy has a notebook and a strategy ready and waiting. And you say his family is supportive. He'll be fine now.'

The consultant had told me that working with Tourette's patients would be satisfying, and it was. But I had spent over six months here and it was time to go. This clinic was my last stop in general child psychiatry before I qualified and started forensic work with young people.

My journey through childhood disorders had been interesting and perhaps more demanding than I had expected. Generally speaking, I found it harder to diagnose a child than an adult. Of course, the disorders might be the same: it is possible for children to suffer from bipolar affective disorder, be depressed, or have gestating personality difficulties and even show signs of psychopathy. The procedure to follow when diagnosing might also be the same: the starting point is most likely the International Classification of Diseases. This is a manual containing clinically relevant lists of symptoms and most doctors use it. But people are unique and rarely fit into neat categories, and this is especially true of children. I found they very often had a whole constellation of symptoms which could turn any list on its head. And there is something important to remember when diagnosing: the young brain is still developing and changing, so a label that might stick to and stigmatize a child for years would be inappropriate. There are ways of saying that a young person might, just might, grow into psychopathy, without actually calling them a psychopath right now.

I had learned a lot by the time I qualified in general child psychiatry. I thought then that children were very interesting and complicated. But I was about to find out that children who commit crime are still more demanding.

18

I soon started to notice that children in the criminal justice system tended to have very different parents from children in the health system. Parents who were more middle-class, or anyway highly articulate, tended to seek a diagnosis for their child's behaviour and these were the children I had been seeing in the health system. Those who wound up in the criminal justice system very often had parents who could not fight for them. Perhaps because they did not know how. Or because they could barely manage their own lives, let alone their children's.

On one hand it was depressing, because there was nothing I could do about the poverty and deprivation that seemed to characterize so many of the families I was now meeting. On the other hand, making a difference, even a small difference, could go a long way for a child in trouble.

Josh was one of my first cases. His notes were surprising. Nearly all of the children I was assessing forensically arrived with an extensive bundle, often from the police, social services, school, youth offending teams and sometimes the local Child and Adolescent Mental Health Service. Often I wondered how someone so young could amass quite so many notes. Not Josh, though. He did have a few notes. But they related to a single offence.

He had set fire to a chemistry lab. It had been quickly

evacuated but not quickly enough: the fire had spread to a corridor where a few children had become trapped. All had been frightened and one had been rushed to hospital, his face and upper body badly burned. Luckily he had not actually died, but he would very obviously bear the scars for the rest of his life.

Josh had made a sort of firebomb using an aerosol can and a lighter and he claimed that this had simply been an experiment. The school chemistry lab is, of course, the place for experiments – but controlled experiments, because it also contains some highly flammable substances. Had Josh chosen the lab for his firebomb so that he could inflict maximum damage? The school certainly did not believe that the firebomb had been intended as a harmless experiment. The head teacher had called the police, and the victim's angry family was pressing charges. Now the court had asked for forensic psychiatric reports.

Josh came with his grandfather. His grandmother was at work today, and so were both his parents. His grandparents looked after Josh and his younger brother during the week. The boys went to their home after school and either their grandmother or, more often, their retired grandfather, was always there.

I was impressed by him the moment he walked in. He brought with him a sense of calm. In fact, he showed every evidence of a healthy relationship with his grandson. Not too distant but not too enmeshed, kind and caring, focused on Josh but not over-focused. I remembered my own grandfather. Parenting may falter for all sorts of reasons, but a child will probably stay safe if an outstanding grandparent is on hand. So, what had gone wrong for Josh?

He was only eleven and had just started at secondary school, but he was huge: he could have been mistaken for a boy four or even five years older. I had to keep reminding myself of Josh's age and it helped that his grandfather firmly held his hand at the start of the interview. He seemed to want and need that.

The school notes said that he had become a bully, picking on much smaller kids and, significantly, occasionally threatening them with a cigarette lighter. Apart from their size, he apparently chose his victims at random. He didn't even know most of them. This gave me a strong indication that his bullying was not about focused anger. Was it more about fire?

I thought about the boy whose life had been changed by Josh's action, disfigured forever, doomed to explain his appearance by telling and retelling the story of Josh and the firebomb all his life. As an adult forensic psychiatrist, I had struggled to stop myself thinking about the victims of my patients' crimes. And yet, I had to avoid that trap. It was essential to work completely objectively. My mind must be emptied of emotion so that I could be both curious and perceptive. Now the victim was a child, I found myself struggling still more not to be ruled by the emotions victims can arouse.

'Would you prefer Grandad to stay, Josh?' I asked him. He sat very still, his face a blank. No sign of the swaggering, fire-throwing child the school had described. He was more like some small night creature, astonished and terrified in the car headlights. I turned to his grandfather.

'Would you mind staying for a bit, Mr Leadbetter?'

I knew what his reply would be. He squeezed Josh's

hand tightly. 'Not at all, Doctor, I'll stay here if you're up for that, Josh?'

Looking a bit more relaxed, Josh nodded.

I had already learned to treat child patients with respect. Not to face them with a barrage of questions they were expected to answer, as if they had been hauled up before the head teacher. But to make them feel they had some control over the interview. To let them know that their feelings mattered to me.

'I know it's difficult, Josh,' I began, 'but we do need to talk about what happened at school with the aerosol can. Would that be okay?'

No response. He didn't even look at me.

'As you know, I've been asked to speak about this in court, so it's really important. I'll be asking what sort of things you were thinking. Is that all right?'

Still nothing. I had to ask myself if Josh's silence was a response to something I was doing. The clinic was running a bit late: was I showing my anxiety about that? Was I hurrying him by speaking too quickly myself?

I decided to slow right down. I would speak in a more measured, calm, reassuring way – a bit like his grandfather, in fact. And I would minimize my body language and be still. Through my voice and body I would try to signal that it was all right to speak to me and that I was giving him the space to do that.

'So . . . I read about what happened. I was wondering what was going through your mind when you made the firebomb. Can you remember what you were thinking at the time?'

He shook his head. Slightly. It wasn't much, but it was something.

'This must be difficult to speak about,' I said sympathetically and now he gave a small nod.

'Sorry, I know it's hard, but it's something we have to do. I read that you used an aerosol can and a lighter. Could you tell me where you got them from?'

He glanced rapidly at his grandfather and then said, very quietly: 'Home.'

'From home? Was it your grandad's lighter?'

'No, mine.'

'Yours? You have a lighter?'

He shrugged. I thought we were getting somewhere but there was a danger of retreat now. Time to take the spotlight right off him and let him relax while the focus moved to his grandfather. Knowing when to focus during an interview and when to pull away was a skill it was taking me a working life to develop. I already knew that the process worked best when the interviewee felt in control. I wanted Josh to create space around himself when he needed that.

'Do you mind if I speak to your grandad about the lighter?' I asked Josh now. 'Would that be okay?'

He nodded and looked relieved.

'Do you know where Josh got that lighter from?' I asked Mr Leadbetter.

'He loves lighters, he can't get enough of them, can you Josh? Other children sit staring at a screen, Josh sits staring at a lighter. Flicking it on and off, on and off. No use taking his lighters away, he just gets another one. Not hard, is it? They're ten a penny these days.'

I glanced at Josh and he was smiling, very slightly, as if even the thought of lighters gave him pleasure. Evidently he found them exciting and, although he was only eleven, I had to consider the possibility that this was sexual excitement. The occasional association between fire setting and sexual arousal cannot be ignored.

'What do you think, Josh?' I asked. 'Why do you like lighters so much?'

He shrugged.

'How do they make you feel? Happy?'

He nodded.

'Was that the first time you'd taken a lighter to school?'

'I'd sometimes taken one before.'

A whole sentence! This was progress.

'So, why do you think that was?'

'I dunno, I just like them, in my pocket. The plastic and that? Feels nice?'

The longest sentence yet, and an enlightening one. I stayed calm and relaxed.

'So, you just like the feel of them? The plastic and the metal ends and that little round wheel thing? Or do you actually like the flame?'

'All of it, I like everything about them.'

'So how long have you liked them so much?'

'Dunno. Ages.' He looked at his grandfather. 'Years and years?' It was a question.

'A couple of years, I'd say, love,' his grandad said.

'Have you ever started any fires at home, Josh?'

He shook his head. 'I just watch the flame.'

'So, why did you take the aerosol can into school that day?'

'I didn't. It belonged to Craig, he's in year nine. He let me play with it and showed me a couple of YouTubes.'

This was the first I'd heard of Craig and his aerosol can and his YouTube videos. His name had not appeared in the school notes or the police reports.

'That very day?'

'Yeah. Rad vids, with flames and that. So yeah, I tried it in the lab, that's where Craig said it would work best.'

'Did you mean to hurt anyone?' I asked.

Josh shook his head with a new vigour.

'Have you started any fires since that day?'

'No, never.'

But now the grandfather spoke up.

'Sorry Josh, love . . . you haven't started any fires but you still play with lighters. I have to tell the doctor that. He needs to know that you just can't seem to stop.'

'I see. So can you remember when you first became interested in fire?' I asked Josh.

'Dunno.' He looked at his hands.

John Brontë and I had discussed fire setters. It was an interest we shared. We had agreed that it was important to learn the historical context, because past behaviours do tend to predict future ones. But how could that apply to Josh? He had no history of actually starting fires. Just playing with lighters. If I could get to the bottom of this, I might be able to mitigate risk by making Josh more aware of the unconscious drivers of his behaviour. Of course, to do that, I had to work out what the unconscious drivers were.

'Have you ever been hurt by a fire, Josh, in the past?'

'No.'

'Anything in your past at all to do with fire?'

'No.'

'No fires at home? You haven't seen anywhere burnt down, even just through a window?'

'No.'

And now his grandfather spoke. 'Except for the fire at the youth club,' he said. 'Josh doesn't remember that.'

Ping. Something reverberated inside my head. Or maybe it was more physical: a frisson, a shot of adrenalin, a slight shiver. Just occasionally, that feeling told me that here was a breakthrough.

'So, what was the fire at the youth club?' I asked, trying to ensure that my tone remained even.

Mr Leadbetter looked at Josh and then at me.

'It happened about two years ago and it was terrible. The place was well and truly gutted. Josh was hiding in a cupboard when the fire brigade arrived, poor boy. The lads did manage to get him out but they reckoned two minutes more and . . . well, the worst could have happened.'

So Josh had been trapped by fire and it had nearly proved fatal.

'That must have been terrifying. Can't you remember anything, Josh?'

He shook his head and looked down.

'Is this something you two talk about?' I asked Mr Leadbetter.

'Nah. We don't talk about those things, do we, Josh?'

'I'd like to speak a bit about it now. Is that okay?'

Josh nodded. Then he looked up at me and, for the first time, caught my eye. I sensed that this was something he did want to talk about – although he may not have been aware of that need until now.

'How did the fire start?' I asked his grandfather.

'Well, generally people said it was arson. The police told us it was local kids and that it was gang-related. Josh wasn't in a gang, he's not like that, neither are his friends, he was only nine for heaven's sake. But there are a lot of gangs around our way.'

I turned to Josh. 'Did you know about that? About the gang starting the fire?'

'No.'

'I don't suppose you remember much about the day of the fire?' I asked his grandfather. 'Before youth club, I mean? Do you happen to recall what Josh was doing?'

'Yes, I was just semi-retired then and I was home that day. We had our tea and we were watching videos – your nan was there, wasn't she, Josh? We had a routine, Josh likes routine. So Tuesdays it was school, home, tea, telly, youth club.'

'Was it the same routine after the fire?'

'No, it stopped when he was out of hospital. He was there a few days with smoke inhalation and when he came home he just stopped with the telly.'

'What do you think you were watching that day, Josh?'

There was a long pause. Not a stubborn pause or a painful pause, definitely a thinking pause.

'*Minder*!' he said suddenly, smiling, looking pleased. He had retrieved a memory.

'*Minder*! The TV show from the eighties?' I was surprised.

Grandad had smiled at the word *Minder* too. There was remembered pleasure on both their faces.

'Yes, Doctor, that old series! See, we had a VCR machine and we had lots of old videos that Josh's dad recorded because he loved that programme. Then we'd watch them with Josh and his brother. They're even better the second time around and Josh really enjoyed them.' His face fell. 'But the VCR's kaput now.'

'Can you remember the episode you watched that night?'

More thinking. I watched Josh's face change as he remembered.

'Yeah, I remember! I was watching it and . . . and . . .'

Who would have guessed that *Minder*, of all things, could give Josh a key to his traumatic memory?

'. . . and then the fireman pulled me out of the cupboard and carried me outside. Yeah! It was freezing cold out there!' He looked amazed at himself. He had reached inside and found something which trauma had taken away for two years.

We were quiet and still while Josh thought. I could almost see him replaying the memories. Or was I projecting that? I only know that our silence felt precious, like a starting point that might take him to a healthier place. When he eventually left the room, he walked taller and he had lost that empty, blank look.

I finished the assessment. Fire setting is surprisingly common among young people: it is highly risky and it taps into something ancient and human in all of us. That fascination with flames and their danger so many of us feel must date back to our ancestors. But the young fire setter sees something more in the flames.

So many of the antisocial and dangerous behaviours of young people are about control – and fire can be an attempt to control the external environment, forcing others or the world to behave as the fire setter wishes.

Of course, it's not that straightforward. Because the young fire setter has the control to create mayhem – but no power to control it once created. The use of accelerant can give an illusion of control. Until it simply leads to a more rampaging fire which destroys all in its path and which may not be stoppable.

John Brontë and I had shared the theory that this ultimate lack of control, this impotence in the face of absolute natural power, resonates with some young people. Perhaps there is a parallel with a violent family home where the young are helpless in the face of physical and emotional abuse. Starting a fire reframes that experience of helplessness into something of their own making – which may give them back an element of power, or anyway the illusion, for a while, of control.

There was no such theorizing in my report about Josh. He came from a poor home but certainly not an abusing one. And he was not exactly a fire setter. But I did believe I had uncovered the cause of his obsession with lighters. I referred him to the Child and Adolescent Mental Health Service but I also arranged to meet him one more time. I believed I had developed a genuine, empathic connection with him: children know when your empathy is fake and I felt I had earned Josh's trust. He had been given some food for thought, so a bit of time for reflection before another session might help him remember more.

It did. The second time I saw him he was able to talk in depth about the fire and his interest in lighters. Finally, I said: 'Josh, I've given you a lot of thought since I saw you last. I do think you may be scared of fire, deep down.'

He stared at me but said nothing.

'When something like that happens, it can be really upsetting. And being upset by fire can make you scared and more interested in fire at the same time. I think that certainly happened to you, because I don't believe you had even picked up a lighter before the fire at the youth club?'

He nodded agreement.

'How do you feel when you click on the flame?'

He looked defensive. 'I don't feel scared.'

'I can see you get a lot of satisfaction from lighters. But I think that deep down you're scared of the flame. So maybe the real satisfaction comes not when you flick it on. But when you flick it off.'

His eyes were fixed on me.

'Because that means you can control the fire. You couldn't control that terrible fire at the youth club, but you can control the flame on a lighter which you've started yourself.'

His grandfather had been sitting silently throughout. Now he frowned and leaned forward.

'You think it's about turning the flame *off*, Doctor?'

'Yes. I think it's about the fear you have, Josh, very deep down, of fire. A totally understandable fear. Lighters please you. They please you a lot, because you can use one to turn off the flame.'

Forensic medicine is busy and perhaps too busy. I would have liked the luxury of reaching this sort of revelation with a patient slowly, over a series of therapeutic sessions, but my workload did not allow that. I just had to lob the idea at Josh and hope that he ran with it.

A few months later, his local CAMHS contacted me.

'It's about Josh. He's lost interest in lighters! Completely!'

I felt something inside me whoosh up towards my head. That sensation of pure pleasure at good news.

'That's wonderful! What work did you do with him?'

'We knew all about the fire, everyone around our way remembers it. The blaze was horrific and I remember how people were saying a child had been found in a cupboard and was only just alive. So we knew how traumatized he must be. We did some trauma-based work with him and then sent him to the London Fire Brigade, as you recommended.'

The Fire Brigade runs a very good course for juvenile fire setters – the trick is to ensure that the young person is in a psychological place to benefit from it. If they're in the wrong place, then they will just reject it. And, when he was first referred, Josh had refused to attend. So the psychological sessions used that as a starting point and, after a month of regular sessions, he had built up the confidence to join the fire course. From there he was flying.

'It all worked, Duncan! He simply has no interest in lighters any more.'

I hope I haven't made Josh's case sound as though dealing with arsonists is simple. I'd worked with a few in high-security units and I knew only too well what a catastrophic effect fire can have on the psyche. Many cannot recover from it. And maybe Josh recovered only because he was so young at the time of the fire and had received the right interventions.

This early case brought me especial pleasure. Here was the very reason I had moved into child forensic psychiatry. I had wanted to intervene early enough in young lives to change their course and that's just what had happened to Josh. All those years of training felt vindicated and for a while the world was a benign place. That didn't last long. In fact, it stopped as soon as I met Callum.

19

'You are a dickhead,' Callum informed me. 'Did you hear me, dickhead?'

Callum was just fifteen and, after an argument with an elderly neighbour, had severely battered the man. The boy's solicitor, Will, was someone I had dealt with before and had thought good at his job. He had now contacted me for my help in defending Callum.

'Certainly mitigating circumstances here,' Will had assured me. 'The court needs to know about Callum's problems, how his ADHD has ruined his life.'

I was visiting the boy in the home of his new foster carer. We were in the living room, the foster carer and I in armchairs and Callum sprawled across a sofa at such an oblique angle that he was almost turning his back to me. He was wearing a hoodie and the hood was up, so that I could see little if anything of his face. His body told me that he was a big and sprawling lad.

'Callum, would you mind taking your hood down a bit?' I requested politely.

'Nope.'

'I would prefer to see your face.'

'I don't care.'

I changed direction.

'So, you've just had a birthday. How did you celebrate?'

He did not reply but fished his phone from his pocket and started texting.

Was I irritated? Oh yes. And I could have told him in no uncertain terms to take the hood down. But that would have ruined any hope of engagement. It was more productive to examine my own feelings to help me understand what might be going on for him. Not to show my irritation, or be biased by it, but simply to use it to try to understand and be more curious. So I let him text his friends while the seconds ticked away and his internal world started to unspool in front of me.

A guffaw. A grunt. Callum did not take his eyes off his phone and soon his fingers were tapping intensely again. Another guffaw. I watched his interaction with his phone as he snickered and then sighed.

I observed but I did not respond. A young person speaks with every shrug, every gesture. And silence allows them a sort of voice. Their communication may be non-verbal but the only way to get anywhere near the truth is to let them use the voice they have chosen. Even if that voice consists of snickers and grunts and clicks. Even if it is intensely annoying.

Callum's ADHD had been diagnosed only two years ago. He had refused to take any medication for it. About a year later, he had attacked his mother and, for her safety, he had been removed from the family home. He was placed in care and there he was violent to other children, and so he was moved once more, this time to a secure unit. I was interested to learn that he had thrived in this enclosed environment. But, on release, he had beaten up his mother again. She was not pressing charges. However, the neighbour who was attacked soon afterwards by Callum felt differently; he certainly wanted the boy charged. Callum was currently living on bail with his new foster carer.

There were a lot of social workers and others scratching their heads about this boy: just what should they do with him? This question was soon to be asked in court.

The foster carer seemed both kind and brave in her dealings with such a big, violent boy. She explained now, in answer to my question about his birthday: 'Callum couldn't go out to celebrate because he's living under bail conditions.'

'I see. Do you have any mental health difficulties or issues, Callum?'

He continued to ignore me. Perhaps he guessed I already knew the answer to that, but anyway his foster carer supplied it.

'Callum's been diagnosed with ADHD.'

'Thank you,' I said gently, smiling at her. I turned back to Callum. 'But I really need to hear it from Callum.'

Silence descended – apart from the tapping of fingers on phone. After a while, the foster carer began to shift uncomfortably in her seat. Silence can be agonizing but I do believe that it is essential if a child is to have any voice at all.

Soon, Callum stopped texting and put down his phone as though it bored him. He sat, his face hidden, his body very still.

The boredom might have been an indication of ADHD but I could discern no other symptoms. I could not fully assess him in a one-off meeting like this, but I was far from certain he really had ADHD.

'Have you taken medication for ADHD?' I asked him.

'I don't know.'

'You must know if you've taken medication or not?'

'I don't take medication, I'm not going to fucking take any medication. People want me to take fucking pills but I am not taking fucking pills. Got it, dickhead?'

I gave no indication whether I'd got it or not. I was waiting, pausing, to let the temperature drop a little. There would be no hope of a useful meeting if I met his aggression with aggression – it simply would have turned into a contest, Callum versus me. I let his aggression drift away.

'So. How do you like to spend your time when you're not at school?'

'I don't go to school.'

'Are you in alternative education?'

'No.'

'How do you like to spend your time?'

'Get out with my mates.'

'How many friends do you think you have? Roughly?'

'I don't know, you spaz, I don't count them, do I?'

An insult. I felt its sting. That word again, spaz, the word I had heard all my childhood – shouted across the playground, sometimes shouted by adults in the street; anyone at all might suddenly shout spaz when they saw my mother. It still had a powerful, almost dizzying, effect on me. As though my blood had stopped circulating and had decided to go around the other way.

I sat very still and quietly, trying not to show any emotion, suspecting that Callum knew he had scored a bullseye. But when I looked up, he was tucked inside his hoodie, playing on his phone. I breathed deeply. It was clear to me that Callum had no boundaries, and not just in this room but in life, too. I decided to put down a boundary. I would insert a little authority to see how he might react.

'What did you just call me?'

'Spaz. Dickhead. It's what you are, I already told you that. Spaz dickhead.'

He wrapped his hoodie even more tightly around his face and started to snigger into his phone. But I knew these insults could not be brushed off. They had to be registered, by Callum and by me. This time I decided to let him know his words had landed.

'That's not helpful, Callum. I'm here to make a report for the court. Do you understand the importance of that?'

'I don't care.'

'So you don't want to speak to me?'

'I don't care.'

'Are you finding this interview stressful?'

'No.'

'Some people believe that you should be placed on a community order – how would you feel about that?'

'Yeah well, that's not going to happen.'

'You would rather go to prison, then?'

'Yup.'

'Why is that?'

'I don't know.'

'Do you watch TV or go to the movies at all?'

'No.'

'Do you ever listen to music?'

'No.'

'What do you do on your phone?'

'TikTok.'

'Could you rate your mood out of ten, where ten is really happy and zero is –'

He turned and looked at me for the first time. His body had been angled away until now and it was a shock to see, suddenly, his plump, smooth face close to mine, bristling with fury. This was an intimidating young man and I did not feel safe, but all my instincts told me that I must not show fear. I stared back into his eyes. His pupils were large, as if we were sitting in the dark, and his mouth looked like a knife's gash across his face.

He shouted directly at me, far, far too loudly: 'I don't fucking know.'

Once again, I waited for a moment to let the anger dissipate. I was close to terminating the interview, and if I had been alone in the room with him I would have left. I can examine aggression and anger up to a point, but it is senseless to stay if there is a strong possibility of violence. If he attacked me, it would be bad for both of us.

The foster carer was standing now, pleading with Callum, begging him to calm down. I decided to stick with the interview a bit longer.

'You don't need to shout, Callum. I can hear you.'

He turned away again. After a pause, I continued to ask questions. In answer to almost everything, he said that he didn't know or he didn't care or that I was a spaz or a dickhead.

He only engaged once during the interview.

'How old were you when you first attacked someone else?'

'I don't know.'

But I could see from the way his cheeks bulged and the line of his hoodie changed that he had started to smile.

'I think,' prompted the foster carer carefully, having evidently read the mountain of notes about him, 'that you were nine, almost ten, Callum.'

I asked: 'Did you hurt this person?'

Callum was openly laughing. He didn't look at me, but he let me see his face.

'Yeah, well, I hit him with a fucking fence post, so I reckon he was hurt, yeah.'

'Was it a wooden post?'

'It . . . it was . . .' Callum was spluttering with laughter now. '. . . concrete.'

'Do you think that's funny?'

'Yeah.'

'I'm writing a report for the court, and I'll have to include that.'

'I don't fucking care.'

'How many times do you think you've been arrested in the past?'

Callum started to laugh again. When he was almost rocking in his chair with laughter, he volunteered some information for the first time.

'Let's say, eighteen.'

'You've been arrested eighteen times?'

'Yeah.'

He apparently enjoyed himself during this part of the interview. He soon reverted, however, to his don't knows and don't cares. When I felt there really was no more to be gained from continuing, I stopped. With some relief.

It seemed from his notes as if every doctor, every carer,

every family member and of course every lawyer who had ever voiced an opinion on Callum had consistently, after each crime, pleaded for his release without charges. Everyone insisted that locking him up was not the answer. The consensus view was that Attention Deficit Hyperactivity Disorder was responsible for Callum's actions, not Callum, and that if he could be persuaded to take medication for this, everything would change.

To have committed so many crimes and to have persuaded so many people that these were not his fault, well, that was quite a feat. Before I interviewed him, I had wondered if I might meet a boy of profound charm. Obviously, that had not proved to be the case.

'You will write that report soon, won't you, Duncan?' his lawyer said, when I described the interview. I hesitated. Who would not hesitate before working in defence of Callum?

'By the way,' added Will. 'He's given permission now for you to speak to his mother. That's important. She doesn't want to see you; she's agreed you can phone her. I've got the number here.'

During the interview, Callum had effectively refused me this permission. By saying repeatedly: 'I don't fucking care.'

'Look,' Will said, 'he's signed for it now. He does take a while to get to know people, that's why he was so difficult with you.'

Hmmm.

'Duncan, I wouldn't say that engaging with strangers is his strong point. But I hope you were at least able to establish how very traumatic his childhood has been.'

'No, because he wouldn't answer any questions.'

'Good thing you're talking to the mother then, she'll tell you all about it. I really think much of Callum's behaviour can be explained by ADHD and early life trauma.'

'So, Will, which medical school did you train at?'

'Come on, Duncan, it's not rocket science to recognize that the boy acts out because he's traumatized. His father was an extremely violent drunk. Disappeared now, but Callum's behaviour is his father's legacy in my opinion. I think we should consider post-traumatic stress disorder as mitigation for poor Callum's behaviour.'

'Will,' I said awkwardly, 'childhood trauma isn't generally accepted as mitigation for a series of such violent crimes.'

'Not alongside the ADHD?'

'I struggled to find evidence for that.'

'He's been diagnosed, I can confirm it, we'll get the medical records to you in the next couple of days.'

It is essential to check medical records – whatever impression you might have of a young person in the room. Who knows why they behave the way they behave? Factors like pride, fear, anxiety, all these might distort a doctor's perception. The medical records are collateral evidence and a cross-reference.

Will said: 'I think you'll find that the mother sheds a lot of light on things for you. I'll get her number today.'

20

Callum's mother was expecting my call and answered on the very first ring. That sounded like an energetic thing to do, but from the moment she greeted me I could hear exhaustion in her voice. I wondered if her exhaustion had set in long ago, when she was coping with a younger Callum and a violent husband. And there was a daughter too: she had been born three years after Callum.

'Callum's solicitor has suggested I ask you about his early years,' I said.

She explained that his father had left when the boy was five. He had certainly both experienced violence himself and witnessed violence towards her. It had all ended with his father's departure.

Clearly Callum had internalized the violence, identifying with the aggressor. Some children who are abused – sexually, physically – internalize trauma; they identify with the victim and gravitate towards self-harm. Often, they find themselves in the healthcare system. Others, who externalize damage or identify with the aggressor, may find their way to the criminal justice system. There are also children who fluctuate, and their pendulum can swing backwards and forwards between violence to self and violence to others, and so backwards and forwards between the embrace of healthcare and the strong arm of the law.

But Callum was, I felt, clearly heading towards a future in just one place: the criminal justice system.

'You know, Doctor, he can be a bit rough when he gets upset about things, but he's a sweet boy underneath it all,' his mother insisted.

'It's hard for me to tell, because he simply wouldn't engage with me.'

'Well, he doesn't with new people.'

'Why do you think he gets into so much trouble?'

'Oh, he's got ADHD. Definitely. I've seen it in others and I know. And underneath, Callum's a very anxious child. I understand anxiety because I suffer from depression myself.'

'Do you think he feels any remorse for attacking your neighbour?'

'No. He was provoked and he had good reason really, because our neighbour is a very rude man. He said some nasty things to Callum.'

I imagined that quite a lot of people had wanted to say nasty things to Callum. Including me when he had kept calling me a spaz and a dickhead.

I said: 'He told me he's been arrested eighteen times.'

'Oh dear. Well, I wouldn't be surprised.'

'Do you think he was doing that sort of thing for a good reason eighteen times?'

'Well, a lot of times maybe.'

'Does he ever show remorse?'

'No, he doesn't.'

'So, how do you explain his behaviour?'

'I think having ADHD doesn't help, but my own personal opinion is that he's autistic. I wouldn't be surprised if they don't find that out. And of course, some of it's probably caused by anxiety or even depression. Did I tell you that I suffer from depression myself?'

Callum's mother had offered me a fairly full catalogue of the conditions and disorders which are often proposed to excuse criminal behaviour. Not to mention the early childhood trauma that Will the solicitor thought should be included.

I spoke to Callum's foster carer, but she said that he had been there too short a time for her to make useful comments.

'Although,' she added, 'I did notice how, during your interview, Callum was really enthusiastic when he talked about his previous violence.'

I agreed with her.

'Do you think you could persuade him to take his ADHD medication?'

'I've tried. He's not going to do it. I wish he would, it might change everything.'

Finally, I spoke to his probation officer.

'It was quite difficult to interview Callum,' I told her.

She chuckled.

'Welcome to my world.'

'So he's always difficult?'

'He can never really express any feelings about anything. His standard response is: "I don't care. Fuck off."'

'I got: "I don't care, fuck off, you dickhead."' I couldn't make myself say spaz.

'Yup, sounds like Callum.'

'His mum thinks he's on the autistic spectrum.'

'His mum is surprisingly dismissive about his violence,

considering she's often his victim. We have certainly tried to assess him for autism, but we can't unless he engages with us.'

'How often do you see him?'

'An hour a week.'

I wondered what it would be like seeing Callum for an hour a week. I doubted the probation officer looked forward to it.

'I wouldn't say we get any useful, structured work done together. Because it's always on his terms. He talks a bit about what he's been doing, that's all.'

'There seem to be a lot of people arguing that he should stay in the community.'

'Well . . . I have to say that he's the most dangerous kid I've ever worked with. I do expect him to kill someone sooner or later.'

'So you think he should go back to the secure unit?'

She sighed. 'Errrrr . . . he was only there a very short time. Maybe they should try to make him take his medication first . . . you know, if he could just be treated for his ADHD . . .'

'Have you seen medication work for really dangerous kids with ADHD before?' I asked.

'I'm not sure. But it's certainly worth a try with Callum.'

'You don't think he should be locked up again?'

'Not yet. I think it would be better to treat his ADHD and give him a community order. The secure unit must be a last resort.'

I thought of Benjamin, the first child I had seen with ADHD. The boy who had been on the point of exclusion because the teacher could not cope had turned into one of the brightest kids in the class simply by taking amphetamine salts. I had argued and fought against their use, but once I had seen their effect I had become an advocate. Of course, I could not help hoping that the change I had seen in Benjamin might be replicated in Callum. I knew that ADHD had found its way from the health service and the education service into the criminal justice system by now. We are, as a society, anxious to forgive children and reluctant to criminalize them. I was no exception.

'Listen,' said Will. 'I think I can get the court to agree to suspend Callum's sentence or just give him a community order on the condition that he takes his medication. But I'll need you to say it will be a gamechanger. And of course, I'll explain to Callum that this is his last chance. We may have a completely new kid!'

'I will need to be sure of his ADHD diagnosis,' I said.

'Okay, sorry for the delay; we'll get the medical records to you today, I promise.'

Despite the fact that Callum had been given eighteen last chances already, I agreed to advocate that he should have another. Amphetamine salts had worked like a miracle in an educational context. I wanted, no, needed, to believe that this medication might work in a criminal context too. I reminded myself that the probation officer had said the medication could change Callum, despite branding him her most dangerous client. We all wanted it to work.

This was exactly why I had chosen to focus on child psychiatry: my hope that things might change. Callum presented with antisocial behaviour (also called conduct disorder) as well as ADHD and, after studying his notes, I believed he did fall into the category of children who can be diagnosed with hyperkinetic conduct disorder.

I liked this therapeutically hopeful diagnosis. It meant there was a chance that ADHD medication could change his behaviour. Think of the conduct disorder as a raging fire and the ADHD as lighter fluid, making the fire that much more uncontrollable. Treating the ADHD could mean that the young person would be less impulsive; it would give them a little more time in the moment to make better decisions.

There was one other hope attached to this: a diagnosis of a mental disorder can give some young people a face-saving way to change. Accepting an illness and taking medication can externalize bad behaviours and enable better choices. I had never seen that happen in a child as violent as Callum. But I decided it was worth a try.

And so, fuelled by hope, the report I wrote for the court suggested that Callum's behaviour might, just might, be significantly changed with the right medication. Of course, the court, too, wanted to believe that there was an explanation for Callum's violence, that the explanation was medical and that medicine would solve the problem.

I did air the possibility that the ADHD diagnosis should be confirmed again and that the drugs should be initially administered during a stay in a secure unit. This latter suggestion was ignored by the court, where it was decided he should receive a community order and a nineteenth chance.

I heard no more for some time. I thought that the amphetamine salts must have worked.

21

One pleasure my new specialization brought was that I could sometimes work with John Brontë. He had agreed to be my supervisor for the first really major homicide I handled as a child and adolescent forensic psychiatrist. I was to defend a sixteen-year-old boy called Thomas in the Old Bailey. I was nervous. Because Thomas was a rare sixteen-year-old. He was a serial killer.

Thick iron bars obstructing a patch of natural light, concrete walls, plastic chairs, a defendant sitting behind a metal table which is dead-bolted to the floor – prison interview rooms are nearly all the same. John Brontë sat slightly to one side, watching as I questioned Thomas for an hour.

This boy was not at all what I had been expecting. After studying his police and medical notes, I had developed assumptions, something I hope I have since learned not to do. I had thought he would be like the many gang members I had interviewed: a big lad, or at least a wiry, tough lad, who would initially present aggressively, nonchalantly, even disdainfully.

Instead, Thomas was small for his age. He was thin with wispy blond hair and a baby face. I could not imagine him roaming the mean streets. And I certainly could not imagine him killing three people, nor compiling the kill list which had been found in his school locker.

He answered my questions quietly. Sometimes he looked at me, but his eyes also tended to roam around the room. After a while, I noticed that he kept glancing anxiously at the same place. It was behind us and directly between John and me. He seemed to do this covertly. He was certainly very quick. Only if I looked up suddenly from my notes would I catch him. It happened once, twice. The third time, I began to develop an almost irrepressible urge to turn around. Just what was he looking at?

Eventually I gave in to this urge. But, of course, there was nothing there. Only more concrete wall.

I felt the hairs on the back of my neck stand up. It really seemed that Thomas could see something in the room that no one else knew was there.

Thomas had killed three men by an unusual method: sticking a screwdriver into their heads. Specifically, their ears. And he had been caught with a screwdriver while allegedly stalking his fourth victim. He had already admitted to his crimes, although he claimed not to remember actually committing them.

Unusually for a child who kills, his victims were adults. In fact, they were all men. They had not been known to him but they had not been chosen entirely at random either. It seemed that he picked his victims out quite deliberately: in queues or on the street or in shops; anywhere he could study them first. Then he followed them, choosing his moment to kill them. I had occasionally encountered similar behaviour by gang members undergoing initiation rites. I questioned Thomas quite intensively about his friendships. And it was obvious there was no gang. He operated entirely alone.

John and I had been sure that his victims must all have something in common apart from their gender. We had both studied the file intensely. We could find nothing. They were different heights, different colours, different ages.

The police had been convinced he must have some connection with his victims. They had searched Thomas's home, his bedroom and his school locker for information in vain. But among the items they had found in the locker was his sinister list. On it were the names of students at his school (and in fact one teacher) whom Thomas planned to kill. The police knew this because he had helpfully labelled it 'My Kill List'.

Perhaps many angry children secretly harbour such a list, not really intending to do anything about it. I had certainly already encountered a few. In each case, our forensic service had been contacted by the school which had found the list, perhaps after episodes of violence or bullying.

Curiously, these were usually private schools and the compilers of the lists tended to be white, middle-class teenage boys. Such a boy had not long ago confided to me that he had 'practised' for the list by actually killing someone: a homeless man no one would miss. I assumed this to be a fantasy but the strength of his conviction worried me. He described in forensic detail how he had chosen the place – a forlorn and lonely patch of mud under a bridge – and how he had lured his victim there. Breaking confidentiality when a crime is suspected is not something any psychiatrist can take lightly. With great reluctance and good advice, I finally decided to contact the police. They searched the area and did indeed find a body. So now I was a great deal less inclined to dismiss kill lists as fantasy.

Thomas's kill list was a very unusual one because, try as they might, the school could fathom no reason for the names on it. Some of his projected victims were virtually unknown to him. None were in his class or any other recognizable membership group and no one on the list could recall any incident with Thomas of anger or harm. It appeared, like the men he selected as his victims, to be an entirely random list.

I asked Thomas now about My Kill List.

'It was nothing,' said Thomas.

'Was it like a game? Or something you thought you really might do?'

Thomas glanced rapidly and surreptitiously at that same spot on the wall.

'I thought maybe I would,' he said.

'But I suppose you didn't expect to get very far down the list. You probably guessed you would have been stopped after you'd killed the very first person.'

I was trying to sound reasonable, as if we were simply discussing homework or some normal adult–child topic.

'I didn't think,' said Thomas, 'that anyone would ever guess it was me.'

It was true that this small, childish lad was not someone you would easily suspect of such a crime. At my side, I felt John nodding. I was glad he was there, glad I had such a talented senior clinician to mentor me through my child forensic work. Sometimes I wondered if one factor in my decision to train in this specialization was that, subconsciously, I had wanted a chance to work more closely with John.

'So . . .' I said. '. . . I was just wondering about the screwdriver?'

He looked at me and then, disconcertingly, glanced very rapidly to that place behind me again, his eyes quickly returning to mine. Once again, I felt the hairs on the back of my neck lift a little.

'You told us you weren't carrying the screwdriver to use as a weapon when the police arrested you, so I'm wondering why you had it with you in the shopping centre? Sorry if I missed that, could you explain it again?'

He stared at me now and gently chewed his lower lip. He looked mildly perplexed. John was watching him too and I was sure we were both thinking the same thing.

Being perplexed isn't exactly the same as being confused; it's more than that. There's a sense of bewilderment, of disordered thinking, of someone trying to make sense of the world and almost succeeding but not quite. I have seen it very often and it is connected to various disorders. I remembered seeing it on the face of the first patient I ever detained under the Mental Health Act, Petra. And that is where I had subsequently seen it most often: on the faces of psychotic patients.

I wondered if I would get a 'no comment' to my question, as the police had. But he gave me a little more.

'I just happened to have it.'

No matter how many psychiatry textbooks are written about it, truthfulness is something that can only be judged at the time, and the best judge is experience. A large proportion of forensic patients do lie to the psychiatrist, but by now I liked to think my antenna could pick up falsehoods. Was Thomas lying? Did he really not know why he had the screwdriver and what he would do with it?

'It's a strange thing to carry,' I said casually. 'Can you think of any reason you might have had it with you?'

He shook his head. Not because he couldn't think of a reason but to indicate that this was all beyond him somehow.

John gave me a glance and I think he was telling me to tread carefully. The records of psychiatric interviews can be scrutinized, so there's no hiding anything the defendant has said. And if, for instance, a different account of the incident is given from the account given to the police, then the psychiatric expert witness is wading through deep ethical water. On the other hand, asking the defendant about their health or psychological difficulties can and does mean they might suddenly open up – and that can have a helpful impact on the case.

'You mentioned earlier that you hear voices . . .' Another can of worms here. An astonishing number of offenders hear voices if they think voices can shorten their prison term.

And now Thomas seemed keen to talk about voices. He nodded with something like vigour.

'When did you last hear them?' I asked.

'Today.'

And then it happened again. That rapid glance behind me, more precisely, over my shoulder, so swift that I almost missed it. Afterwards, Thomas's face resumed its intense, fixed stare.

I asked: 'When today?'

Another glance, another intense stare.

I was cautious: 'Thomas, do you see something back there?'

I had already fallen into the trap of looking once; I wasn't going to do it again, even though I wanted to. That would have felt collusive. But it did really seem something must be there. Even just a picture on the wall. Although I knew there was nothing.

'No,' he said. And he immediately broke eye contact, staring down at his fingers.

'Are you okay?' I asked gently.

He looked back at me and nodded. His eyes flicked over my shoulder for a fraction of a second, and then stared again at his hand, where his first finger was tapping against the ball of his thumb. Were these random taps? Or was there a rhythm, or something anyway that might have significance for Thomas? I listened carefully and could discern nothing.

And then, to my surprise, he spoke unprompted.

22

Blinking a little, as he continued to look down at his hand, Thomas said rapidly: 'He's in here.'

His voice was so quiet that at first I wasn't sure I had heard him. I waited. He said nothing more. Finally I asked: 'Who's in here?'

'The grey man.'

Ah, the grey man. An old friend of mine. He pops up in interviews with defendants of all ages and he is nearly always grey, although occasionally he is green. I have never actually seen him because only the defendant can do that. His role has usually been to instruct the defendant to commit that crime.

It is hard not to greet the grey man's arrival in an interview with scepticism, but I try not to. And especially not this time. Just to make sure, I glanced at John Brontë and supposed his hair was sort of grey. Although more white really. And I was showing a few signs of grey. Although more brown really.

And then I did it, the thing I shouldn't do. I looked over my shoulder. Just in case there was someone there because, unless Thomas was a brilliant actor, I was sure he really believed there was.

'He's here in the room with us?' I asked.

He nodded.

I did not point out that the wall was blank. I took him

seriously and perhaps that was why Thomas seemed keener to engage with me now. If a patient is having a real auditory or visual hallucination, then whatever they see is as real to them as anything actually in the room. I thought suddenly of the horror films I used to watch as a teenager. Oh, what a classic situation. A young boy, two cynical psychiatrists and, unseen by them, a grey man standing, watching silently in the corner . . .

I made sure my voice was low and gentle. 'What are you seeing back there, Thomas?'

'Him.'

'Does he have a name?'

He gave a small shake of the head, hardly moving. He was not snatching rapid glimpses at the grey man now but looking openly at him for longer.

'Have you seen him before?'

He replied with intensity. 'Every day. All the time.'

'Does he speak to you?'

'Sometimes.'

'What does he say?'

'He tells me to do stuff.' He stared down at his fingers again. The tapping stopped. He began twisting his thumb instead. 'Bad stuff.'

'What sort of stuff? Could you give us an example?'

'Like the screwdriver, stuff like that.'

'So what did he tell you to do with the screwdriver?'

But Thomas had stopped talking and was looking anxious, shifting in his chair.

I persisted. 'Did the grey man tell you to kill those people, Thomas?'

He did not reply and I knew I should pull back.

'Do you ever hear him speak when you don't actually see him?'

There was a pause.

'Yeah, a lot of times. Mostly I don't see him when he speaks. And when I see him, he just looks at me.' Thomas was talking quickly, in an undertone. As though confiding – or even as if he didn't want the grey man to hear.

'His voice, is it clear like mine is right now, or is it muffled?'

'Clear. Like yours.'

I waited for him to say more. He did not.

'So . . . is his voice inside your head?' I asked gently. 'Or is it outside, right in the room?'

This is a key question for some psychiatrists who are trying to judge whether a patient really does hear voices. Personally, I take each case in context and will listen to either answer, but there are psychiatrists who, if Thomas had given any other reply, would be entirely convinced he was not telling the truth.

'In the room. Like yours.'

'So, it sounds real, his voice?'

He nodded.

I didn't even have to look at John to guess that we both thought the same thing. Thomas was psychotic. Not acutely – he wasn't presenting us with stories about how he had just finished a phone call with the President of the United States. No, his speech was relatively ordered and everything he said made sense, well, at least it had a rationality of its own.

I'd trained for adult psychiatry in a lot of jails, where people were frequently unreliable narrators, and by now I knew that it's the small, subtle indicators that often point at the truth. The way Thomas glanced furtively over my shoulder, the stare, the tapping on his hand, the perplexed look, all had helped to persuade me that he believed what he was saying.

I asked him if he ever experienced anything unusual, and he looked baffled.

'I mean, like thoughts being put into your head, or taken out? Or perhaps your body not being under your own control?'

He shook his head.

'Do you ever feel as though anyone is watching or following you outside? Or maybe they are in your room?'

'Yeah, in my room.'

'What happens there?'

'Well, sometimes people watch me – not the grey man. I mean, he does. But other people too.'

I asked him to tell me more.

'Not here. At home. The wall is sometimes like, liquid. Like liquid glass. And people see through it, they watch me through the liquid.'

'And can you see them?'

He became forlorn.

'I try to, but when I look it turns back into a wall.'

'So . . . what do you make of that? The wall and the liquid?'

He had no answer.

Every child should have a safe place to retreat to: this is a fundamental need. But many do not. In their own spaces, they often face real life threats: of violence, perhaps, or abuse. And a boy like Thomas who imagines he is being watched can feel threatened in the same way. He can feel there is no boundary to keep him safe, that there is no escape.

I asked another question.

'Do you ever see something which you think is really important, something which other people don't seem to notice at all?'

He replied at once.

'Yeah, keys. My mum's keys.'

'What do you notice about them?'

'So, when she gets in and puts down her keys, they're always pointing to this picture of me on the shelf.'

'Like . . . a school photo?'

'Yeah, it's a school photo, she really loves it and she keeps it on the shelf. So her keys always point at that picture. Always.'

'What do you think that means?'

'Sending me a message.'

'What message?'

He did not reply. He just shrugged.

'Something about the grey man?'

He shrugged again. Maybe the grey man. Maybe not. The world was a perplexing place for Thomas and he didn't have the answers.

The keys were what we call an idea of reference: that is when someone sees significance in an event which is more likely to have occurred by chance. It is a useful indicator of an underlying or emerging psychotic illness. As a forensic psychiatrist for adults, I had sometimes tried to explain this in court to juries. But often they just didn't get it. Hallucinations, screaming, phone calls via Mars with Elvis

Presley who was not dead but hiding in East Lothian: that was the sort of psychosis juries seemed to prefer, not the subtle symptoms. In Thomas's case, it was his very subtlety that convinced me he deserved a robust defence in court.

There was one other thing the jury would be asking themselves. I knew that because I was asking it too. I took a breath and plunged in.

'Thomas, there's something else I'd like to speak to you about . . . is that okay?'

He gave a small nod.

'It's about the screwdriver. I know you don't remember exactly what happened when you used it, but I'd like to ask you something about the men. I mean, the men who died. I'm sorry to do this, because I know it's hard for you, but could we speak about that?'

I did realize that I was on shaky ground but, since we already had enough to make a case, I thought it was worth taking the risk that Thomas would shut down completely now. I watched him, waiting for him to freeze.

But he didn't. He nodded again and then swallowed. He had already agreed that he had killed three times but added that he had no memory of this. True memory loss after killing someone is a controversial area. Homicide is, after all, a psychologically significant event. It is traumatizing not just for the ante-mortem victim and for the victim's family, but also for those who actually carry out a homicide. Yes, most murderers do inflict trauma on themselves. So you might expect them to retain some memory of it.

In Thomas's case, I saw his alleged memory loss as an important scaffold for him – holding his life and psyche in place while he underwent investigation and legal scrutiny.

As his assessing psychiatrist, I had no intention of pulling his safety scaffold away. Although I was ready for the prosecution to try doing just that.

'Thomas . . . it seems you killed three people by pushing the screwdriver into their ear. And I'm wondering . . . why into the ear?'

A pause. Thomas looked around the room. I had not expected him to answer and it seemed he would not. Then suddenly he said, as if it was obvious: 'Because of the noise.'

'The noise?' This was confusing. Did he mean the voice? 'What noise?'

'All this! All the noise!' His voice was louder now.

'But . . . I can't hear any noise. What do you hear?'

'Buzzing, droning, whispering. On and on. It has to stop, it has to. He tells me that.'

At my side, I felt John Brontë leaning forward slightly.

'Who tells you that?' I persisted. 'The grey man?'

Thomas nodded. 'So that's why.'

'Because of the noise? How long have you been hearing it?'

'Quite a while.'

So he had been sticking screwdrivers in his victims' ears to stop the noise. I sat for a moment in reflection. Because I did understand noise in the ear and how it could drive you crazy. The torment caused by the fistula inside my own head had only ended a few years ago and I would never forget it. Thomas's psychological symptoms could have been as miserable for him as my physiological disorder had been for me.

I said: 'I totally understand why you would want to stop

the noise. Totally. But I don't see why you had to kill people to do that.'

He did not reply. In fact, whatever I tried asking him now received no reply. He had stopped talking. So we sat in a silence he did not break. I was thinking that, after all this time, I was no nearer understanding why this small slip of a boy had turned into a serial killer. Or why he had harboured a list of future victims. I glanced at John and his expression told me that he had no theories either.

We reached the end of our allotted time and a prison officer came in to take Thomas back to his cell. He left calmly, without looking at us.

We collected John's old car from the car park. Once we were safely inside it, we turned to each other.

I said: 'I really think he was seeing someone who was standing just behind us. It spooked me, actually. When the hairs on the back of my neck stand up, it usually means the offender isn't acting.'

John started the car. 'That perplexed look. That wasn't acting either.'

'And the liquid wall!'

We both nodded.

'Definitely psychotic,' we said.

23

We had a shock when, at the case conference, his barrister showed us a different Thomas on CCTV footage.

A police bodycam had recorded the boy's arrest on a busy street. You could see the public gathering in the background, staring, shocked, curious, as paramedics persuaded them away from the ambulance. Thomas did not look surprised as he was handcuffed, and he did not resist. The officer half-chanted his rights and Thomas said: 'Yeah.' He was asked questions but he simply shrugged in response. He looked nonchalant. Not psychotic.

The next footage was recorded soon afterwards at his police interview. Again, he mostly gave no comment, but it was his body language that was so striking.

An arrest on a murder charge would be enough to crush most of us. Not Thomas. In this footage, he was initially a sulky, defiant teenager, shoulders hunched, the son you wish your friend hadn't brought along to the picnic. Then he slouched back in his chair, arms crossed behind his head, legs stretched out far in front of him, one ankle over the other. This was not so much the defiant teenager as the annoyed passenger delayed at an airport and trying to get some sleep. What Thomas didn't look like was a sixteen-year-old who had just been arrested on a murder charge.

'You're the experts,' said the barrister, 'but frankly this isn't my idea of how people behave when they're psychotic.'

It was true that nothing we'd picked up from the mousy kid in prison was present here. This boy was not perplexed or anxious and if he thought the grey man was there, he did not glance at him. For the first time I had to ask myself seriously if he could have been acting when we saw him in prison. Surely not. I looked at John and he shook his head. No, of course Thomas had not been acting.

'I agree it's hard to see there,' I said to the barrister. 'But the boy we met in jail has prodromal psychosis, at the very least. That means the psychosis may only just be emerging.'

The barrister continued to look sceptical and I didn't blame her.

'It was the subtlety that convinced us,' I added.

'Well, if you're confident, I'm more than happy to run that defence. But I'm really not sure that subtlety will cut it, not for the judge and certainly not for the jury.'

'I think we should go for manslaughter with diminished responsibility on the grounds of psychosis,' I said. 'I really believe that's true. Thomas isn't insane but he has an emerging psychosis that would have significantly impeded his decision-making ability at the time of the offences. Alleged offences.'

'Don't worry about alleged, there's too much evidence for that. But what about intent? Could he form the necessary intent to harm, if not kill?'

I said: 'I think he intended to cause harm at the very least. But his mental disorder did impair his decision-making and I believe he needs medical help.'

And so I found myself nervously preparing to take the witness stand.

John tried to reassure me. 'You know, even the most experienced expert witnesses feel anxious. It's normal.'

I took comfort from two thoughts. First, that the room was full of fellow humans and, if I stumbled or my cheeks burned, the jury must simply recognize our common humanity.

Second, that I would be flexible. John had told me that to give evidence I should emulate a Japanese skyscraper. They are built to sway a little in an earthquake. A rigid structure is the first to crack under pressure. So I should concede sometimes, but remain strong on the points which mattered.

I felt ready. Until I watched the prosecution's psychiatrist on the stand. Concise, polished and extremely convincing, she spoke with the great ease of the highly experienced witness.

Did she agree with Dr Harding's report that the defendant was suffering from an emerging psychotic illness? No, she did not.

Did she agree that the defendant was suffering from a mental disorder that had an impact on his ability to make sound decisions at the time of the homicides? No, absolutely not.

How did she explain what could only be described as the defendant's bizarre killing behaviour, if the defendant was not suffering from a mental illness? She could not explain it, not within the framework of mental disorder as understood and manualized in the International Classification of Diseases, Version Ten, anyway.

But surely, behaviour like this must represent mental illness? No, not necessarily.

Then how else might one explain the defendant's actions? Well, simply, that he had decided to kill – and did so. Some things could not be understood within a social construct, certainly not within a construct of mental disorder. Some people were just evil and no further explanation was possible.

Evil. I winced at the word. But the psychiatrist was charismatic. Eloquent. Her presentation of evidence was robust. I watched as the jury melted. Here was an expert witness with a stamp of authority, a woman they felt they could trust. Our defence barrister had a go at her but she remained unflappable.

My heart sank. I stepped up to the stand and, sure enough, it took the prosecution barrister just minutes to make mincemeat of me.

'So, Dr Harding, it seems that a person can kill at random, leaving bereavement and mayhem in their wake, then be interviewed by you, say they hear voices and . . . lo and behold! They are no longer culpable!'

I opened my mouth to reply but the barrister was enjoying himself and determined to hold the floor.

'Mention a few voices and it's a game changer!'

'He didn't mention voices, he responded to what he heard.' That was lame and it did nothing to impede the barrister.

'A defendant only has to say he hears someone who is not in the room and he no longer has to take responsibility for murdering three people! That's right, isn't it?'

He had stopped at last. I swallowed.

'No. That's not right. I have never suggested that anyone who hears voices should be exonerated if they have killed someone. I have to consider each case separately, and in Thomas's case I became convinced that here is a young person showing symptoms of an emerging psychotic illness. Hearing voices was part of that, but . . . well, I mean . . . there were other signs and symptoms.'

Too hesitant. Too vague at the end. I could feel my collar tightening. I wished my face didn't redden so easily. I tried to remind myself that, when I stumbled, the jury would recognize our common humanity. What a daft idea that seemed now. One glance told me I was simply losing them.

'Emerging? You are saying this illness has not yet emerged?'

'There are some symptoms present now. Hallucinations, for example. But emerging, or prodromal, means that we are seeing signs and symptoms of an illness that is still developing. I am a child and adult psychiatrist and often use these phrases when talking about children because, when we see psychosis start to emerge in childhood, we may well be seeing the first signs of a chronic mental health disorder which could endure into adulthood.'

Better. But of course the barrister looked unimpressed. Worse, so did the jury. The barrister shuffled his papers and the court waited. I knew it was all for effect: the jury, captivated, focused on his every move.

He looked up at last.

'Dr Harding, if the defendant really was suffering from the chronic and enduring mental disorder that you describe, surely he could still form the intent to kill another person? And then actually make the decision to kill?'

'Yes.' I didn't like it, but I had to admit it.

'Yes,' he repeated. 'Yes. A person who is psychotic can still be a murderer. But this defendant is suffering from an *emerging* psychotic illness! He is not even psychotic – by your own admission!'

'As I explained –'

'Yes, you did explain!' The barrister nodded a skilful apology at the judge for cutting me off. 'But how can we agree with you? How can we agree that the defendant should be mitigated from his responsibility for killing three people because he *may* be experiencing some "*emerging symptoms*"?' He used the phrase as if it were a dirty dish-cloth he had found in someone else's sink. 'Thank you, Dr Harding. I have no further questions for this witness.'

I stood in the box feeling helpless. In fact, feeling naked. The prosecution had just removed my clothes.

It was time for our defence barrister to question me. Could we salvage the situation?

She took a moment to shuffle through her notes and then looked at me reassuringly.

'Dr Harding, you told us today that the defendant is suffering symptoms of a prodromal psychotic illness, an emerging illness as you further explained. How might such an illness impact on the functioning of the defendant? I mean, in his daily life?'

I drew breath.

'It could have a catastrophic effect on a young person's ability to function. And, in my view, the defendant's symptoms have pervaded every aspect of his life. He was anxious, paranoid and experienced perceptual abnormalities. That is, he saw and heard unusual things daily, voices that commanded him to act in a certain way: it is impossible to live normally in these circumstances.'

'Do you think he was suffering from these symptoms at the time of the alleged offences?'

'I think that is the case.' I heard my own voice. I sounded pompous. Why couldn't I stand here and just talk to the jury the way I would talk to someone in a cafe? Explain things in an accessible way without dumbing down?

'Thank you,' she said, smiling kindly. 'And do you have any thoughts or theories about the unusual method of killing? The defence accepts as a matter of fact that a screwdriver was used. But can you suggest why?'

'I have thought about that; in fact, I did discuss it with the defendant. I believe that he, on some level, found the voices and noises he was hearing distressing, perhaps unbearable. The pathologist has shown that he destroyed the ear canal of his victims. I think this was connected to the voices he himself was hearing. He believed they were instructing him to do this. But perhaps he was also showing that he did not want to hear them – in fact, perhaps he was trying to stop the voices.'

'And your report says that you believe the defendant's responsibility for the killings is diminished, is that right?'

'Yes. In my opinion, with voices in his ear and the strong suspicion that he was being watched, he could not form a rational judgement. He may have killed those men, but in my opinion he did not murder them. He killed because he is unwell.'

The defence had no further questions and I thankfully stepped down from the witness box. As I took my seat, I looked straight in front of me, not to right or left. Just like a defendant. And I couldn't help feeling that I had been on trial myself. One small mercy was that there were no journalists here to record my humiliation, tapping away on their laptops. Because of Thomas's age, the judge was strict: no reporting of any kind.

When the jury was sent off, John Brontë and I quickly found our way through security to the cells below. I felt sure Thomas would accuse me of performing badly and letting him down.

But when we found him, he looked surprisingly relaxed, stretching his legs out, his arms crossed behind his head again, but this time like a satisfied company director receiving this quarter's results. We stared. This was not the perplexed and mousy boy we had interviewed in jail. This was the Thomas we had seen in the police recordings.

'Thomas . . . ?' I began.

He did not greet us. He barely turned towards us.

'I am so fed up,' he announced. 'It's the way they say it.'

A murder charge is likely to make anyone fed up, but the reason Thomas gave was not coherent. I looked at John to see if he had understood. He had not.

I asked: 'Was it something your own barrister said?'

'Her and the bloke, both of them.'

'Which barrister said what?' John asked, looking confused.

'All of them said it. Every single person in that court.'

'Said what?'

'Defendant. The defendant! That's what they keep calling me. Defendant this, defendant that. Why don't they say what I really am?'

He sat up straight now, uncrossed his arms and slammed his fist into his palm.

John and I glanced at each other in confusion. I wondered for a moment whether we were witnessing a psychotic breakdown. Could it be that Thomas's prodromal psychosis was evolving right now into fully fledged psychosis?

But a part of me suspected something else. Something which made me feel very uncomfortable after the evidence I had just given on the witness stand. I suspected that Thomas was not psychotic at all.

We both stared at him. His eyes small, his mouth big.

'I mean,' he demanded, 'why don't they just fucking say it?'

'Er . . . say what?' I asked.

'Serial killer!'

'But –' began John.

'They should stop calling me the defendant and start calling me a serial killer! Why can't they do that? Why? Why?'

There was a silence.

'Serial killer?' I echoed at last. 'That wouldn't help your defence at all, Thomas.'

His arms opened wide. 'That's what I am! An important fucking serial killer!'

John and I did not look at each other but I believe we understood the same thing at the same moment. That Thomas was railing against a lack of notoriety. He was furious at the absence of a spotlight. Upset by a perceived slight against his agency in all of this. He had killed three people and had a list of many more potential victims. And he wanted to be famous for it. The court reporting restrictions had not been protecting a minor as far as he was concerned. They had stood between him and notoriety.

I thought about that camera footage from the time of his arrest: when the police had asked him about plunging a screwdriver into his victims' ears, he had shrugged in an airy and uncaring way. Here was the beginning of an awful feeling. That we had been wrong about Thomas.

The jury was not out for long. Its members rapidly found him guilty of murder. And it seemed to me now that they might be right.

John Brontë was philosophical in the pub afterwards.

'Bad, mad, bad, mad,' he mumbled into his whisky. 'Maybe Thomas was bad, but there is no question that he was mad as well. I really don't like the way the courts want someone to be mad *or* bad when we very well know it is possible to be both. Psychiatry is not the black-and-white, open-and-shut science that juries want it to be. Why do we study the complexities of the human condition for years if everyone then ignores them?'

'You still think we were right about the psychosis?'

'Oh, I'm sure we were right.'

'He wasn't just . . .' I could hardly say it. 'He wasn't just . . . acting?'

I really believed that I was experienced enough to know the difference between a boy who was actually mentally disordered and a boy who was pretending to be. Any number of adult offenders had tested their acting skills on me over the years and I liked to think I wasn't fooled. As for John, he had spent a long career assessing, specifically, children. Surely, we had not both been hoodwinked by a teenager?

'No, there was definitely an emerging psychosis there,' he said now. 'I'll put money on Thomas finding his way into a secure hospital within six months.'

I decided that this was a case I would keep an eye on. I looked around at the busy pub. Standing room only. There were lots of people from the law courts in here, discussing cases, discussing football, discussing each other. The real world. It is always a shock to encounter it when you've been buried in a case.

John said: 'The biggest danger of a diagnosis, any diagnosis, is that a mad and bad offender receives treatment for the mad part of them. Problem solved! He's been treated, he must be well now and he won't commit any more crime! As long as he takes his medication, they'll believe they've fixed him. He'll be released, because he's no longer mad. But guess what? He's still bad! He buys another screwdriver and he's off again!'

I shut my eyes.

'I became a child forensic psychiatrist because I thought there was a chance of righting whatever's gone wrong for children before they become adults,' I said. 'And now you're telling me that some children are just bad. Did you hear the prosecution psychiatrist describe Thomas as evil? She did, John, but I never use that word and I don't want to believe that's true.'

John looked at me kindly.

'You've had a horrible time. We've all been roasted on the witness stand at some point, and we all hate it. But we do heal, Duncan. However, you've learned enough for one day. This is not the time or place to discuss evil.'

24

We left the pub: John turned west and I turned east. The wind almost blew me up the street. Litter and leaves swirled in the paths of buses, people wrapped their coats around them, umbrellas flipped inside out. It was exhilarating to be outside in busy central London. I thought of the northern housing estates where I had lived as a boy, the very opposite of this colourful, vibrant world. Lights were appearing now, in the street, in the shops. Their warm glow made me think of home and my pace quickened.

'Duncan! Good evening!'

A tall, bearded man had halted in the crowd. Captain Haddock! The hospital and the law courts were very near each other and the professor who had masterminded my fistula treatment years ago was on his way home from work right now. During all the time I had been a fascinating case, we had got to know each other quite well. Getting to know Captain Haddock was one of the few pluses of being fascinating.

We exchanged pleasantries.

'No sign of any further vascular build-up?' he asked curiously. He had predicted that the fistula beneath my brain's dural membrane might gradually rebuild in another part of my head. 'No throbbing?'

'None. All I have at the moment is some anger about the cause of it all.'

He raised his eyebrows.

'Really? What did we agree was the cause?'

'Head trauma when I was a kid. And I don't think I ever really told you, but I believe it must have been because my dad punched me so much.'

We had halted in the middle of the pavement and people flowed around us. The professor wrinkled his face so that his mouth disappeared for a moment inside his beard.

'Your father's punches must have caused many problems, Duncan, but I don't think your fistula is likely to have been one of them.'

Suddenly, in this street of movement, I was very still.

'But I thought . . . ?'

'I recall having quite a long discussion about the cause with your surgeon. Didn't I tell you about it?'

Nope. He had not told me about it.

'Well, as you know, all those arteries built up around a blood clot which had been there for a long time. And according to your surgeon, the clot may have been spontaneous. But it was much more likely to have been caused by severe childhood illness rather than a blow or an accident. Didn't I ask you about that?'

On my left was a bus, laden with people, staring ahead of them as if they were all driving it. On my right, a pub: HAPPY HOUR ENDS AT 6 TONIGHT SO HURRY, HURRY, HURRY FOR HAPPINESS! And in front of me, Captain Haddock. Giving me what felt like devastating news.

I opened my mouth to reply, but he was ahead of me. 'So, did you in fact have a severe childhood illness?'

I nodded.

'Ah,' he said, 'how old were you?'

'Twelve, thirteen.'

'And what exactly was the illness?'

I did not know what to say. My mouth opened and then closed again. He looked concerned and then gestured to the pub into which you were supposed to hurry for happiness.

'Let's go in here,' he suggested. 'I'm very keen to know more about what caused your strange problem.'

He turned, and I followed him inside. We found a small, cramped table in a corner.

'What was your childhood illness?' he asked.

'Well, I never really knew. I was about twelve and I woke up with a blinding headache one day. Nothing normal. Even opening my eyes made me sick. Whatever it was, I didn't go back to school for a year.'

'A year! But . . . what did the doctors say?'

'For a long time, there weren't any doctors.'

The professor raised his huge, bushy eyebrows.

After my parents' divorce, Mum had lived in fear that my father would persuade a judge that she was too disabled to look after me. When I became so ill, she was scared to call a doctor, in case they involved social services. Who might take me away from her.

It was many months before the school finally insisted that I saw a consultant.

My mother took me to the hospital. I was very weak and very white. A child who had been living in a cave.

The consultant examined me and then turned to face my mother directly. 'Duncan's been gravely ill.'

Mum felt the need to defend herself. She started to

concede that I had been a bit poorly. But the doctor cut her words short.

'I don't know what he's had – some sort of encephalitis. That's an inflammation of the brain. Or perhaps viral meningitis. Either way, it's no wonder his head ached so much. I believe that it was a medical emergency and that it required intensive treatment.'

He paused. He intended my mother to hear his words and feel ashamed. He was telling her off. I wanted to defend her, to explain that she was scared: of Dad, of doctors, of social services. But I was too tired to open my mouth. I looked at Mum and saw that her face was reddening.

'However,' said the doctor, his tone more upbeat now, 'let us rejoice, because Duncan seems to have avoided the worst outcome.'

I wondered what the worst outcome could be. Perhaps some people's heads exploded.

'He's had no treatment and I'm sorry to say that his post-viral condition is now severe. Let us hope there are no later-life complications.'

I will never forget how my mother hung her head then. It was unbearable. My angry, fighting mum. And, for probably the first time ever, she was speechless. She often refused to speak to people, her head high, her mouth a tight, straight line. But now she could not speak. Her face was crimson.

I remember how I sat in the consultant's office and wanted to cry. Not for me but for my mother. I stopped my tears by promising myself I would never, ever blame her for anything, certainly not for this illness, the way the doctor was blaming her now.

'Well,' said Captain Haddock, raising his glass. 'Now we know how your fistula started. Your consultant back then said he thought it was a virus. I'd put my money on bacterial meningitis or encephalitis. Antibiotics would have sorted it out if only your mother had . . .' His voice trailed away. He understood it was wise to go no further. 'Anyway, we know it must have been a severe and untreated brain infection and I'm afraid that many years later you are paying for that.'

'There's one upside,' I said. 'That's when I taught myself to play the guitar. I really got into music during the year I was off school. It's been an important part of my life.'

The professor nodded kindly. 'I'm glad there's a silver lining.'

He asked more questions about my mother and I heard my own answers, drearily familiar. Callipers and crutches. Motability vehicles. Yes, she had a mobility scooter but she'd only used it once. A white Vauxhall now. Moved south. First with me, now in a home counties bungalow. Yes, I spoke to her daily and visited her often.

It was hard to adjust to the knowledge that it was my mother's and not my father's fault I had developed the fistula. I would certainly spare her from this information. Because even the most loving and well-meaning of parents can make terrible mistakes. I knew that only too well. Grandad, whom I regarded as perfect in every way, had made one terrible mistake, many years ago, and my mother could never truly forgive him. She had told me when I was small, after school in front of the fire, in those snatched minutes before we braced ourselves for Dad's return.

When she was three, she said, blowing smoke above my head, Grandad had taken her to the swimming pool. It was there that she had caught polio. The disease had made one leg shorter than the other.

We sat, quietly and solemnly in the firelight, me staring at her strange, redundant limbs. You could hardly tell that one was longer than the other; they were both like rubber hoses. And it was all Grandad's fault.

I loved him so much that I didn't want anything to be his fault. My mother could never hug me or hold me, there was too much metal in the way. Grandad was the one who wrapped his arms around me, bringing both kindness and safety to my life. And he was always the same, not nice one minute and angry the next. He would never have punched me the way Dad did.

I said to the fire: 'Are you sure you got polio at the swimming pool?'

'Yes, I'm sure.' Her voice was harsh. 'I was born in 1947. There was a huge wave of polio soon afterwards and everyone was warned about it. People were told not to go to swimming pools because it was in the water. But your grandad didn't listen.'

I winced.

She put on Grandad's voice, making him sound old and foolish. 'There's nothing wrong with our pools up here in Bishop's Auckland, polio's for those softies down south. Get yerself in the water, love!'

That didn't sound like Grandad at all.

'Then why didn't Grandad get polio, or Auntie Pam or Uncle Billie?' My voice was squeaky. 'Didn't they go in the water too?'

'We all went in the water but I was the only one who caught it.'

She lifted her cigarette to her face. Her mouth tugged on it, fiercely, angrily. 'Then the vaccine came in a few years later. Too late for me.'

I was quiet for a long time. Then I said: 'It's not fair.'

'It's just the way it is. I've paid for your grandad's foolishness all my life.'

And now I was grown up and I had paid for my mother's foolishness with a major brain operation. Perhaps more than one, as the professor obviously expected to see me again in his surgery. But I was determined not to blame my mother the way she had blamed Grandad. I had determined all those years ago, in the consultant's room, that the blaming was going to stop right here.

The professor and I parted company at the tube station, bidding each other a friendly farewell. I was keen to get home. I was in love.

The girlfriend who had lived with me through my fistula misery was long gone. There had been other girlfriends since, and then . . . no one. A few years on my own felt like a necessary part of my journey, but this had ended when I met Hazel. We'd been at a psychiatry conference where, once seminars were over in the evening, musical psychiatrists were encouraged to perform. I had played. Then she had. Watching her, I had fallen in love. It was so simple. Hazel played guitar and composed her own songs and so did I, and soon we were composing a song together. Now we were planning to marry and had decided that the music should be the soundtrack to our wedding.

Our lives together were harmonious. However, we did

share one deep anxiety. For completely different reasons, we were not sure that we wanted to have children. For me, there was a horror that I might turn into my own father. And, professionally immersed in a world of violence, I was tortured by the possibility that I might not be able to keep our child safe. Now there was a new worry to add. Have children and they could blame you for your mistakes for the rest of your life, the rest of their lives. Another good reason to avoid reproduction. No children for me.

At home the flat was warm and peaceful. Hazel exudes calm wherever she goes. I broke our agreement, which is that we don't discuss our work, and told her what had happened to Thomas in court. I shared all my doubts about my earlier diagnosis and together we discussed whether Thomas could really have been feigning psychosis.

But I did not tell her that I had seen the professor. Although she had met me after the operation on the dural fistula, Hazel of course knew all about it. She would have understood my shock and confusion at learning that it was not my father's blows but my mother's fears that had created the problem all those years ago. She might have wondered why I had been so angry when I believed my father had caused the problem and so forgiving when I was told it was my mother's fault. I would need to process that slowly. For now, I could not shake off the feeling that, despite the medical context of our discussion, by revealing my mother's errors to Captain Haddock, I had betrayed her. I did not want to betray her to Hazel as well.

25

I was fully qualified as a child and adolescent psychiatrist and had started to specialize in forensic work with children when I was offered a chance to join an interesting and fast-moving forensic unit.

This NHS service was a hub for any doctor or other medical staff working with young people who were involved (or looked like they might become involved) in crime. When they needed advice, we were there. On the phone, by email . . . and sometimes in person. I remembered how, years and years ago, John Brontë had told me that his skills were more effectively used by seeing fewer patients himself but advising other doctors how to treat their patients. That hadn't sounded very attractive at the time. Now I was doing the same I realized how busy and stimulating this was. I learned a lot and very fast, because the phone never stopped ringing. And because I saw the most challenging cases myself.

After a very intense few years, I bumped into Ari Good. His eyes narrowed.

'Duncan! Not *still* training? Why, you'll be drawing your pension before you're qualified!'

It was true I was now past forty. But I couldn't imagine a more interesting, rewarding job. A new day might bring anything, from knife-wielding gang members to abused children who themselves had started abusing.

'I'm qualified, but it's true I still feel as if I'm training to work forensically with children, it's so highly specialized. But, Ari, I love this work.'

He nodded patiently.

'Most of us become a consultant just the once; now I wonder what you'll decide you want to do next . . .' He waved his long fingers in the air and started to count my qualifications on them ostentatiously.

I grinned at him.

'I haven't been changing, I've been refining. I'm staying in specialist forensic child and adolescent psychiatry.'

He gave me a warm, wrinkly smile. But his tone was cynical. 'We'll see,' he said. 'We'll see if you decide to stick around more than five minutes.'

I knew he was wrong. I had arrived at my destination. I looked back now and understood I had been heading here all along, even when I hadn't actually known that.

In addition to the hectic unit, I continued to work for the court or solicitors. This gave me a much more detailed level of involvement with certain cases. However, when I was asked to travel to the top of England to interview Amelia, I did not immediately agree. Her defence team had requested a report on her, but I was dealing with so many cases that I felt I could hardly take a day to drive so far and spend so much time with just one child.

'Look,' said her lawyer. 'This is a complex and upsetting case, but I'm telling you that you will find it compelling.'

I hardly knew Julia. How could she possibly be sure that I would find Amelia's case compelling?

'Just read the notes,' she insisted. 'That's all I ask. Read the notes. And then you'll want to help Amelia.'

Reluctantly, I agreed. And it turned out that Julia was right. When I had read the bundle, I could not refuse the instruction. I arranged to see Amelia.

I had almost no family left in the north. My mother had moved into her own retirement bungalow about an hour's drive away from me in London. The struggle to be mobile all her life had taken its toll by now and she had finally agreed to have a wheelchair at home. Her white Motability car waited for her on the driveway but had been used less and less until she had stopped driving it altogether.

'I'm going up to Middlesbrough. Nearby, anyway,' I told her on the phone. 'I haven't been up there for years – it'll be strange to go back.'

She said: 'I'm worried about the cat. I wonder if you could get him some vitamins, Duncan?'

We were not good at talking about the past together.

I drove up the motorway, up, up, up, so far that I wondered if I might just encounter a kid answering to my name. But when I turned off the A1(M), the housing became less dense, then sparse and finally stopped altogether. I was in unfamiliar territory now: green, undulating countryside.

An A road then a B road then a small lane and finally a concrete track. The land on either side sloped gently and sheep were grazing in the fields or lazing against the hedgerows. In the distance, nestling into the landscape, was an attractive stone farmhouse.

But this was no farm. Car-park lights, CCTV, a sophisticated alarm system, locks on the doors, an entrance procedure . . . this was a secure unit. And waiting for me inside was someone accused of murdering two people and attempting to murder a third.

She wore a pink sweatshirt with a picture of a pony across the front. Baggy jeans. Pink socks. Around her neck was a freshly made daisy chain. She was twelve.

The unit manager said: 'This is Amelia.'

Amelia studied me from beneath a solid fringe of brown hair. It was cut just above her eyebrows in a straight line and behind it the rest of her hair was tightly harnessed into a ponytail. She looked much younger than her age.

I smiled at her.

'Hi, Amelia.'

She stared back. There was a brief pause.

'Hi,' she said.

This greeting might have been a small success: I suspected she had been debating whether to speak to me at all.

'Nice badge.' She was wearing a small purple badge which featured the face of an old friend of mine: Dr Who. And the Doctor in the picture was from years ago, from when I was a kid, in fact. I wondered if perhaps the badge had belonged to her father. Her late father. But she did not respond to the delight I took in it, so maybe she had just put it on because she liked the colour.

We sat down and I explained that I would take notes as we talked and then I would write a report on her for the court.

'I'm a doctor and usually when you speak to a doctor it's confidential, but not this time. I have to base my report on what you tell me,' I explained, 'and some of it might be read out in court. Do you give me your permission to talk to you?'

She half nodded but seemed anxious to say something.

I waited for her question and, when it came, it was fired rapidly.

'Are you working for the prosecution?'

No other child has asked me that, before or since. It showed an advanced understanding of the criminal justice system for a twelve-year-old.

I shook my head.

'No. You might be visited by another doctor the police will send. I'm working for your defence and I'm an independent doctor and the prosecution's doctor will be independent too. Your lawyer, Julia, has asked me to write the report.'

She nodded and then looked at the floor. This room was comfortable but sparsely furnished. I was sitting in a fake leather armchair which was already sticking to me and which squeaked a lot when I moved. The rug Amelia was staring at was plain and thin. On the ceiling various monitors flickered.

'So it seems you understand that there's a defence lawyer and a prosecution lawyer,' I said. 'And that usually both ask their own doctors to write reports and answer questions in court. We're called expert witnesses.'

She nodded again and I waited. I could see she was preparing another question. Seeking the right words so that it would come out smoothly. After a pause, she spoke rapidly and fluently.

'So there's two expert witnesses, but you say different things?'

'Well . . .'

'I mean, you're paid to say one thing and the other doctor's paid to say another, is that how it is?'

This girl was clever. And she wasn't even trying to be clever. She'd just been thinking about how courts work and now she had asked a question which pinpointed both the failing and the strength of our criminal justice system.

'It could be that way,' I said. 'There's certainly scope for people to look differently at the same facts, but they wouldn't necessarily do that just because they're paid to think one way or another.'

I have seen forensic pathologists, with their labs and their scalpels and their meticulous scientific analysis, offer a jury two completely different versions of the same facts. In forensic psychiatry's broader science, there is still more scope for interpretation.

Amelia was watching me. I added: 'Speaking personally, whether I'm paid by the defence or the prosecution, I just write exactly what I think.'

She gave me an appraising look and then her eyes wandered to the window. Outside, I heard hens clucking.

Amelia, suddenly and surprisingly, clucked back, mimicking them perfectly. I couldn't help laughing.

'That's pretty good,' I said.

She looked pleased.

'I've been practising since I got here.'

She was a little girl again. The ponytail, the daisy chain, the clothes. I knew the clothes were unlikely to be her own. Had she been offered a selection and chosen these because she wanted to look like a younger child, or perhaps even to be a younger child?

She fingered the daisy chain, very gently so that the tiny flowers did not break.

‘I like your necklace, I know they’re quite difficult to make,’ I said.

Amelia continued to look out of the window. The hens had stopped clucking. They still had not appeared.

‘Fran helped me make it.’

Fran was one of Amelia’s carers. She had shown me in, smiling, offering a cup of tea, telling me a bit about the farmhouse. She had made the situation seem almost normal. Of course, she’d been highly trained to work here in a children’s secure unit. She knew she had to be alert and watchful around Amelia, no matter how relaxed she might seem. And, importantly, she would ensure that Amelia had no access to matches, lighters, accelerants or incendiary materials of any kind.

‘What’s it like here?’ I asked.

‘Okay. The hens are nice.’ She was still staring out of the window, as if she was waiting for the hens to appear in the concrete yard. I looked too. But the hens were silent now and the farmyard remained bare, despite its promise of birds and animals.

Amelia’s fingers had been picking at a large scab on her arm. Now they found their way to Dr Who. She ran a forefinger around and around the edge of his face.

‘Oh, and there’s a sweet pony here, called Monty. I don’t ride him but I like brushing him.’

We chatted about Monty and all the time I was watching her. How her fingers kept returning to the scab on her arm until she’d pulled it off. How she then held up her arm and started to nibble at the place where it had been. There were other scabs in other places which her fingers worried at.

This was just the warm-up, but Amelia was proving easy to talk to. It was often my job to engage the unengageable, so she was a refreshing change. I noticed how sometimes she seemed sharp and grown-up, and sometimes she was a little girl. Not so unusual for a twelve-year-old.

But I knew we'd soon have to talk about something very unusual. I'd read the court bundle. I'd seen the forensic evidence. And I'd watched some CCTV footage taken very soon after the fire which raged through her house and killed two members of her family. Until someone is proven guilty, it is customary, of course, to refer to 'alleged' offences. But where children are concerned 'alleged' often isn't necessary: the question is usually not who but why?

Amelia had most certainly set fire to her house. And the evidence seemed to show that she had intended it to kill her family. If that was so, then the police's murder charge would likely stick – intent, of course, being a key difference between murder and manslaughter. Through careful questioning today, I hoped to find out why she had started the fire. And, most of all, whether she had really intended to kill her family.

'I'm sorry to ask, Amelia, I know this is very difficult for you. But could you tell me about the day it happened? The day of the fire?'

Sooner or later, you have to discuss the offence itself and of course that is dangerous territory. Even the most chatty child, and not many of the children I meet are chatty, is likely to entirely shut down when we get there. They might freeze, fall silent or become violent. I waited to see what Amelia would do.

She paused. She was thinking.

'What about it?' she asked at last. Her voice was not hostile.

'Well, maybe you could tell me what you did that day. I think that it was a Saturday . . . was it sunny outside?'

No response.

'So, can you remember what you did in the morning?'

She answered quickly.

'Went for a walk.'

'How far did you go?'

'Oh, it was a long walk. I took an energy bar and a drink, so I mean, quite long.'

I nodded and my face agreed. Yes, that's quite a long walk.

'Did you take anything else with you?'

'A sweatshirt, in case the weather changed.'

I nodded again. My face said: yes, the weather is certainly changeable.

'Did you enjoy the walk?'

'Well, at first. Maybe I went a bit too far. I got quite tired and I didn't need the sweatshirt, I was really hot. So I put it down on a log and then I sat on it. I listened to the birds. That was nice.'

'And how long did you stay there?'

'I'm not sure. An hour? Maybe even more. Then it was getting late so I decided to go home.'

She wasn't picking or nibbling at her arm scabs now. Perhaps because there was nothing left of them, just red marks where they had once been. But she'd started on the laces of her trainers. One of them was coming unravelled and she tugged on it, digging into it with her thumb nail as if she was still making a daisy chain. And, gradually, she was prising the lace's skeins apart. I watched her and sat quietly in case she wanted to say more, but all her focus was on her trainer.

'Do you remember what time it was when you got home?' I asked. 'Roughly?'

'Probably about five.'

I waited, and this time she continued.

'I know that because it's when Dad feeds the dogs and birds. He's like clockwork. Every day. So, I walk down the driveway and he's out in his shed, standing in the doorway, and we wave to each other. We always wave to each other.'

She was using the present tense. Now that day was fully in the past, maybe she could allow herself to experience it in a way she hadn't at the time. Maybe it would always be in the present tense for her. And she was smiling. As if she'd just seen her father, waving to her from his shed.

'Your dad sounds nice,' I said. She did not reply and gradually the smile faded and her fingers separated another skein of the lace.

'So you live in a farmhouse, right? Do you have a lot of animals there?'

'Not really. We just have a little field and Dad lets a farmer down the road graze some sheep in it. He likes leaning on the gate and talking to the farmer. See, Dad really wants to be a farmer too. But we've only got one field and that's not enough for farming.'

Amelia had been sent to this special unit in the north of England until her case got to court, but she didn't come from this area. In fact, she lived with her family comfortably just outside the M25, where the houses are large and local roads congested with expensive cars. Owning even a little field there must indicate wealth.

'So where does your dad work?'

'He takes the train into London quite often and does boring things. That's what he says.'

I laughed. Amelia smiled.

'You were really fond of your dad, weren't you?' I asked and before I'd even finished the sentence I knew I'd made a big mistake. Amelia had been talking about her father in the present tense. And I'd just placed him firmly in the past. She looked up at me now. Her stare was direct.

'I mean,' I hastily corrected, 'you *are* really fond of him.'

But it was too late. We both knew that. Of course, Amelia was aware that her father was dead. According to the notes, she became hysterical when given the news. Then, for some days, mute. I hoped my mistake wouldn't make her mute again.

Was I being dishonest, talking about her dead father as if he was still alive? I don't think so. I was reflecting back what Amelia had given me. Listening is the most important part of a psychiatrist's job, and I mean really listening. Sometimes the children I work with have never been heard by anyone before. Only by listening can we see the world through their eyes and begin to understand. So if Amelia talked about her father in the present tense, it was vital that he stayed there. And, in a way, he really was present: our parents, long after their deaths, do stay deep inside us until the end of our lives.

The silence between us stretched on. Amelia stopped with the shoelace and found a scab she'd missed on her arm. She could hardly reach it without twisting her body, but her fingers somehow managed to push and pull at its edges.

At last she spoke.

'Of course I'm fond of him,' she said. There was no rancour in her voice, no reprimand. I felt forgiven.

'Tell me more about your dad's shed, Amelia.'

'What do you mean?'

'Well, do you ever spend time in it yourself?'

She looked at me, just for a moment, but said nothing. I persisted.

'It's his space: do you like it there?'

'Yes, it's okay, I suppose.'

Her fingernails kept working at the scab, as if she wanted to erase it. But of course, the more she picked, the more scabs she produced. She was still talking to me, but there had been a change in her. I knew I might have lost her. That would be a disaster for her case. Because, if I didn't listen, then who would?

26

The sun had moved around the farmyard while we were talking. I knew that, not because I could see the sun, but from the shifting shadow of the barn.

I said: 'The police found something in your dad's shed, Amelia.'

I spoke as gently as I could. She worked at the scab. Her notes had not mentioned any self-harming, but I did have to wonder if this was the cause of so many wounds. I might ask Fran afterwards.

I said: 'They found money, quite a lot of money. In a sandwich bag. One of those plastic Ziploc bags.'

Amelia did not respond.

'So . . . did you leave that money in the shed?'

No reply.

'You see, the police say your fingerprints are on the bag. And on the money. So you can't blame them for thinking that you left it there. Did you do that?'

She squirmed. I felt cruel, but I had to do this.

'Sorry, Amelia. I know these questions are difficult.'

She glanced at me for a moment and said, with a note of kindness in her voice: 'It's okay.'

I waited. Then suddenly she sat up straighter and placed her hands on her knees. She looked at me directly.

'The police kept asking me about the bag. But I don't see why the fuss. Yes, it was my bag. Yes, I put it there. So what?'

Because a stash of money prepared for a sudden departure shrieked of intent: intent to kill, intent to run. The money had been found pushed behind a pile of wood. The police could not say how long it had been there and the last thing I wanted now was for Amelia to incriminate herself, but I did need to know why she had filled a bag with £20 notes and then hidden it.

I asked her again.

Silence. Then finally she shrugged. 'Dad gave me this emergency fund. He told me I mustn't spend it, just keep it in case anything happened.'

This was interesting.

'Your father gave you the money?'

'Yes, quite a long time ago.'

'And he told you to keep it in the shed?'

She shrugged again.

'No, he didn't tell me where to keep it.'

'So what sort of emergency was he thinking of?'

Amelia considered this.

'Well, you don't know about emergencies before they happen; they can be things which you've never even thought of.'

Yes, like the weather, emergencies do just happen. I nodded agreement but was careful not to nod too enthusiastically, or move too quickly at all. I knew that it was essential to be a calm, containing and safe presence and that meant showing no emotions of my own.

'Did you think of taking the money with you that night? When you left the house after the fire?'

She reached for another scab and then put her hand back on to her knee, as though she had to keep an eye on it, as though your hand was another thing which, like the weather, you couldn't entirely trust.

'It didn't actually occur to me. But I wasn't really thinking about much at all that night.'

She had told the police this and I was glad that she had given me the same story: any differences had to be noted in my report.

'Do you remember when you put the money there?'

'I can't remember when, but it must have been a while ago.'

'I'm sorry to ask all these questions, Amelia, but there is something else I'd like to know about the shed, if that's okay?'

She looked curious.

'Can you tell me about the petrol?'

'What do you mean?'

'Well, I think you syphoned some petrol from your father's car in the shed . . . ?'

She was silent. I knew she wouldn't give me an answer until I gave her a question.

'So . . . did you take his petrol, Amelia?'

'Yes.'

'You siphoned it from Dad's car?'

'Yes, it tasted awful. I sucked it out of the petrol tank with a tube and then moved it up to the house. That was a few weeks before.'

We both knew before what.

I said: 'I've seen people in the movies sucking petrol out of cars but never in real life. What made you do that?'

'Dad did it once. For the lawnmower.'

'So he was mowing the lawn and he ran out of petrol?'

'No. He couldn't even start because he didn't have any petrol in the mower at all. Mum kept saying the place was like a jungle. So in the end he siphoned some petrol out of the car.'

'Did your mum know?'

Amelia shrugged. 'Why would she care? She just wanted the lawn mown.'

We paused. And then, for perhaps the first time, she spoke spontaneously, unprompted and unquestioned by me.

'It was so hot last summer, do you remember? Dad put the grass in a heap and steam came off it. I put my hand inside the heap and it felt so soft and warm. Oh, and it smelt . . . it smelt wonderful.'

She half closed her eyes. She smiled. It was last summer for her right now, a happier, more innocent time.

'The petrol . . .' I reminded her. She opened her eyes. I had just replaced the smell of freshly mown grass with the stink of fuel. 'I've read your statement. And you said there had been an argument a few weeks before the fire. An argument with your mother, I think? Could you tell me about that? I'm not sure what it has to do with the petrol?'

There was a long pause after such a long question. Not that it was over her head. Pitching questions at the right level is essential and I had learned that each interview required continual assessment of the child's verbal and non-verbal responses. That way I could adjust my delivery, my approach, my language. It was the first step in developing genuine trust. And trust was essential for a child to show me their true self.

I was sure by now that Amelia was very intelligent and

that she was easily capable of understanding my questions. Of course, that didn't mean she would reply. The pause that followed went on a long time. Perhaps she was deciding whether to speak. Or which words to use. I sat, still and quiet, trying to give her the space to think.

Then she said, very softly: 'I lose it sometimes. With my mum. I lose it.'

I left another pause to give her more space – not too long this time, though, in case she lost her flow.

'So . . . what happened?'

Silence. She did not move. Not to pick a scab. Not to caress Dr Who. Not to touch a daisy chain.

'Amelia?'

'I did okay in a school maths test and I was really looking forward to getting home and telling Mum and Dad. I mean, my mark wasn't brilliant, it wasn't an A or anything, but I've missed so much school and maths is only just beginning to make sense. Like it's not total gobbledegook any more.'

She chuckled at the word and mouthed it again silently. Gobbledegook. Gobbledegook. She ran the syllables around her mouth like a candy. Then she stopped and there was silence.

I agreed: 'Maths can feel like . . .' I paused. I didn't want to use gobbledegook. That was her own word and she had savoured it. I said: 'Maths can be tricky.'

But Amelia did not break her silence. I knew I had to tolerate it. However long it lasted. I recalibrated, rearranged myself, heard my chair squeak, felt myself unsticking and sticking to it again. All I could do was relax into the situation and watch where it might go.

It didn't go anywhere.

Finally, after I don't know how long, I could stand it no more.

'So . . . you were saying?' I tried to sound relaxed. Breezy. My tone said: hey, what does the destination matter, when we're enjoying the journey so much?

'I got a C in that test.'

We were off again.

'And C's not brilliant but for me it's pretty good. And that's what Dad said, he said: "Pretty good, Colonel, pretty damn good."'

She giggled.

'He calls you Colonel?'

She nodded.

'Yep, doesn't it sound funny? I know it's a joke but I've never really noticed how funny it is.'

She giggled again, then held up her palm. 'And he gave me a high five.'

She stabbed her hand in the air, giving her father a high five.

'How about your mum? Was she pleased?'

'No. She was already in a bad mood, I could tell that before she even said anything. From the way she was banging plates around in the kitchen. So I lifted the test paper until it was right in front of her, so she had to look, she had to see the score. And she did . . . but not really. Just sort of glanced. And then she goes into a big huff because the porridge from breakfast had got stuck hard on to my bowl and the dishwasher hadn't got it off and she's there scrubbing at it. But it's not my fault, I hate porridge and never eat it, even though she gives it to me every day. It looks like sick. I've told her that but she never listens to me.'

I'd been nodding all the way through this, to encourage her to keep going. And she did.

'So, I say: look, I got a C, not bad, eh? And all she says is: will you please take those muddy shoes off at the door, Amelia? How many times do I need to tell you? And by now she's shouting, well almost. She's saying: I MEAN, HOW MANY TIMES?' Amelia's face had turned into a long, angry shout, her mouth thrust forward.

'So I say: Okay! That's fine! No problem! And I pull my boots off and kick them over the floor towards the door. I really, really wasn't kicking them at her but . . . but . . . well, one boot hit her on the toe. It was an accident, honestly it was. But she screams and yells and drops the porridge bowl and then Jay-Jay starts crying. He's my little brother, he's only one and a bit. So, whenever Jay-Jay starts crying, my mum just totally loses the plot. I mean it. Because if he cries, she always starts crying too!'

I nodded. Don't stop, Amelia.

'So she's flapping around and yelling. Jay-Jay's crying, Dad's trying to calm everything down . . . there's noise everywhere. And everything goes like . . . like a red colour. I try never to cry in front of her, never, so I go storming off. That was it. The whole day was ruined. Everything was ruined.

'I went outside in my socks and sat in the shed for a while. My feet were hurting because of the stones on the drive, they stick in you. Anyway, after a bit, I went back in with the petrol.'

'Why?' I asked.

‘I don’t know. I just did. I took the tube out of the shed which Dad uses for the mower and sucked petrol out of the car into a red bucket. I did swallow some. Horrible. Anyway, I took it inside in the red bucket, and then I poured the petrol around.’

‘Inside the house?’

‘Yes.’

‘Where did you actually pour it?’

‘Into the cracks.’

‘Cracks?’

‘Between the floorboards. In the hallway. And then I went into the living room. The cracks are quite big in the living room and there’s a fancy sort of rug under the window and I covered it too, not really sure why I did that. Then I took the red bucket back outside. And it was so nice out there now. I mean, the evening. It was so quiet and still. The sheep had their heads down in the grass, each had its own shadow. And I felt really calm. Like a sort of zombie calm. Like I was dead and just standing there zombified.’

‘Where were your parents?’

‘Well, they were inside, smelling the petrol everywhere. And when I went back towards the house I could hear Mum. Going . . . absolutely . . . mental.’

She stopped. She was still and quiet, perhaps exhibiting zombie calm. For a moment I thought about the notes I could have been taking, how I had to show the court this child, the way she was right now. But I knew notes must wait. I had to listen, travel with her, try to feel what she felt. I had to focus on every word, movement, inflection.

‘Why did you pour the petrol in the cracks?’

'I'm not sure.'

'And how did you even tip the petrol into the cracks? Surely it went all over the floor?'

'Well, it did a bit. But it went down the cracks as well because I used this little funnel thing which is by the door, it's for watering the small plants. Not the terrarium though, you're not supposed to water them. Did you know that?'

I shook my head.

'It's a jar with plants in, right?'

'Yep, a big jar.'

I wondered, fleetingly, how the plants in the jar could live without water.

'So, why did you want to put the petrol down the cracks?'

She didn't answer. She just shook her head. In the silence that followed I heard someone sigh and it was me. Because everything Amelia had just told me shouted of intention. Intention and planning. In other words, murder.

And yet. It was very hard to believe I was looking at a murderer. I could feel nothing but compassion for her. I was sure there was a lot more to know about this strange, fragile child who was now worrying at some other scab. Her vulnerability touched me deeply. She looked broken. And she was pretty much alone in the world: instead of a parent now, there was a system.

'Amelia, will you tell me what happened next?'

I watched her collect herself. She wasn't preparing to lie; she was preparing to tell the truth. So many of the adults and children I had interviewed were trying to present a different version of themselves, different from the truth. But I was sure this Amelia was completely authentic.

‘So, your mum was furious . . .’ I prompted when she did not speak.

She wrapped her fingers around her Dr Who badge, as if he were a lucky charm.

‘Yeah, she was furious and . . . I totally got it. The smell was really awful. It was so strong it could make you sick. And Jay-Jay was crying, crying, crying and that always tips her over the edge. So, she makes me scrub the floor and take the Persian rug outside. She keeps saying that it’s ruined, and she’s right, it’s really, really ruined. And she’s saying: that’s your favourite spot so what on earth were you thinking? And she’s right, I lie on that rug and read, it’s my favourite spot so what was I thinking? I don’t know. Anyway, it took ages to clean. Like . . . three hours. And even then it still stank of petrol.’

‘What about your dad, what does he say?’

‘I get a big lecture from him and that’s really awful. My mum’s standing there with her arms folded and he’s telling me how disappointed he is. That’s the worst thing.’

‘The disappointment?’

She wrinkled her nose and looked deep in thought.

‘Yeah, that’s it. Dad being disappointed is the worst thing. I went to bed and I was thinking about it. He was saying it over and over again, that he was disappointed in me, that I’d really let him down, that I’d let myself down. I cried myself to sleep, I probably cried all night, I’m not sure. So, anyway. That’s how the petrol thing happened.’

My voice was warm. ‘Thanks, Amelia, for telling me. It was brave of you to say all that. It was a few weeks before, so did the petrol smell go away?’

'Mostly,' she said. 'We had to throw the rug out in the end. But in the house, it wasn't too bad.'

'And did anything else happen between the petrol and the Saturday when you went for a walk?'

'Not much. Mum had a go at me about being sent home from school. That was a few days before. Just the usual shouting and then the silent treatment.'

'Why were you sent home?'

'Got into an argument with a stupid boy at school. He threw my bag over a wall, so I pushed him. They sent us both home.'

I made a mental note to consider this later. Maybe even to discuss it with the school. But I didn't want to be sidetracked now that the discussion was flowing.

'So on the Saturday there's no school and you go for a walk, you arrive back at home, wave at Dad and . . . what happens then?'

'Not a lot.'

'Did you see your mother?'

'Yeah, but she hadn't really spoken to me since the row about being sent home from school. That was probably on the . . .' She thought hard. 'On the Wednesday. We sat down to eat and she made a point of speaking to everyone except me, I mean, she even spoke to Jay-Jay, and she never speaks to him. So, after we'd eaten I just went to bed and read my book.'

'What were you reading?'

She was twelve so I thought she might say Harry Potter. As a Harry Potter reader myself, I had enjoyed many a discussion about Hogwarts while interviewing. But her answer was surprising.

'*The Handmaid's Tale*. It was really good.'

'You were behind in maths but I bet you do well in English,' I said.

She shook her head.

'Not especially, I just like reading.'

I like reading too and I'd read some Atwood, but not *The Handmaid's Tale*. I decided that I would. There was probably nothing incendiary in it, but soon after reading it Amelia had started the fire, so I should check.

'What happened when you put down the book?' I asked.

She closed her eyes. I saw that her fists were clenched tightly shut. I was taking her to a very dark place.

27

The light was different in the room now; it was dimming as it shifted direction with the sun. Amelia's face was changing too. Shadows were appearing. As if she had grown up a little while she talked to me. She looked sad and serious.

'Would you like a break?' I asked.

She shook her head and sat very still. Her eyes were shut and said she was closed for business. And then, suddenly, she opened them. She did not look at me. Instead, she stared down at her fingers, as if they might do the talking. I moved and my chair squeaked. I was trying to look relaxed and not betray my hyper-vigilance at this key point in the interview.

When talking about the offence itself, I was aware that every movement, every inflection, is important, no matter how subtle, because children – adults too – have so many ways of telling you things.

I said: 'I'm really sorry, Amelia. I know how hard this is for you. But I need to hear what you have to say.'

She paused for just one beat.

'I was at the end of the book . . .' She was flipping in an instant from silence to a torrent of words. 'I finished it. I put out the light and went to sleep and then I woke up, I'm not sure why. Didn't need the loo or anything, just woke up. And I still had all my clothes on, even my socks which is weird because I never sleep in my socks, I mean I never do that.'

She had run out of words. I waited. She was struggling. I decided to try distracting her from the terrible, terrifying thing that happened next by asking about an earlier moment.

'When you were reading the book, were you fully dressed? I mean, did you just fall asleep that way?'

'I'm not sure. I would normally get changed into my PJs before reading at bedtime. So, I remember sitting in bed with the book, but I can't remember what I was wearing. Isn't that weird?'

I nodded to encourage her. But she had stopped again. She was like one of those toys with a key in its back that needs constant rewinding.

'Do you remember anything specific? What about your socks, do you remember which socks you were wearing?'

She thought hard.

'Oh, my Peppa Pig socks! Yes, definitely Peppa Pig. I got them a couple of Christmases ago, I hardly ever wear them.'

'So who gave you those socks? Or were they a gift from Santa?'

She smiled at me kindly. Whoops. Of course she was too old for Santa.

'From Auntie Josie. I told her once when I was really little that I liked Peppa Pig, well Georgie Pig to be precise, and she never forgot it. She gets me pig-related stuff every birthday and Christmas: pig hair bands, a pig eggcup, a mug with a pig on it . . .'

'So what happened when you woke up in your Peppa Pig socks?'

'I got up. And went downstairs into the living room. It was dark. And I just stood there for a while. And . . .'

And, nothing. Silence.

'Do you remember what you were thinking then, Amelia?'

She shook her head.

'How about feeling? Do you remember what you were feeling?'

'Just . . . nothing,' she said. 'Nothing at all.'

'So . . . then what happened?' I tried to maintain a soft and gentle voice as we moved to the bleakest place. Aware that I was pushing her there.

'It was very dark. And quite cold. I went to the kitchen, to the drawer where Dad keeps the candles and matches so we can fetch them in a power cut. He's shown us how to find them in the dark. So I did. I found them in the dark.

'I went back to the living room and lit a match and just kind of dropped it on to the floor. It didn't actually fall down a crack, I was kind of hoping it would, but the floor lit up. Immediately! It was so weird. As if I'd just switched on a fire. Then I walked out and shut the door behind me, the living room door, I mean. And I didn't look upstairs, I didn't look anywhere, I went straight to the front door and opened it. My boots were right there. I remembered that the stones would hurt my feet. I thought that I should put my boots on. And . . . well, that was that.'

'You're doing really well and being really brave, thanks Amelia. But I have to ask you to carry on.'

There were none of the non-verbal tics from earlier: no scab picking, no daisy chain or Dr Who touching, no squirming around in her seat. She was still and silent. I wished I could pull her out of the darkness and back into this room, with its clean windows, bright vistas, the possibility of a pony or chicken appearing outside. But for a little while longer I had to stay with this small person in the darkness, the fire, the chaos, the destruction.

'I know how hard this is for you, but it's very important that we talk about it. Why did you light the match, Amelia?'

She didn't respond, so after a few moments I tried again.

'What happened next? After you put on your boots?'

'Yes, I put on my boots and stepped outside and closed the door. I wasn't really thinking about anything. The stones on the drive crunched. I took another step and they crunched again. Then another crunch, then another. And there was this crackling sound behind me. My back was warm. And I just kept crunching forward, one step at a time, down the drive, along the road. I didn't look back. I walked and I walked and the next thing I saw was the blue light. I don't know how they found me, I suppose they just passed me and saw me. And they took me in their car to the police station and I went to sleep and then they took me to the hospital for a check-up. And then they told me about Dad and Jay-Jay. And Mum.'

She stopped speaking. And didn't start again. I sat with her for a long time in silence, knowing that she had finished but still daring to hope for more. Her face was pale and without expression. Her body was still and hunched. She really was closed now.

Amelia might have stopped talking but as I drove away from the farmhouse, I could still hear her small voice inside my head. Back on the main road, there were signs to a local beauty spot. I remembered stopping there once, years before, with my mother. Now I pulled into its busy, late afternoon car park and sat quietly behind the steering wheel.

Families walked past me, making their way to and from their cars, the toilets, the tea room, the woodland walks. Families, in all their complexity. A couple of teenagers trailing behind their parents, looking at their phones. A father, leading the way, his mouth in an angry straight line, mother behind him chivvying two arguing children. Young lovers, walking dreamily hand in hand, not looking at each other, not looking at anyone. A middle-aged couple, suppressing a quarrel in public, hissing loaded words until they reached their car and could raise their voices. I looked with particular interest at a pair pushing a pram with a very small baby asleep in it. They leaned in to the baby as though to a magnet. But did they ever wonder how on earth they would keep their child safe in our cruel world? Did they ever fear what they themselves might do to scar or scare their baby?

'Whenever Jay-Jay starts crying, my mum just totally loses the plot. I mean it. Because if he cries, she always starts crying too!'

I felt as though Amelia was in the car with me, I could hear her voice so clearly. I opened the door and breathed in the warm, summery air.

In the tea room, tired women served a long line of customers. I took my coffee to a distant, shady table outside where crumbs, iced lolly sticks, empty sugar sachets and a highchair, askew, told the story of its previous occupants.

I got out my notes. It had been more important to listen than take notes at times during the interview and I should try to add as much as possible now, while the interview was still fresh in my mind. I drank my coffee slowly until I had finished.

My phone was full of messages. There was a missed call from Amelia's solicitor and I tried to return it but she was out of the office. I made my way back to the car. I wished I could stop hearing Amelia's voice.

I mean, my mark wasn't brilliant, it wasn't an A or anything, but I've missed so much school and maths is only just beginning to make sense.

I heard her all the way back down the motorway. Eventually the lanes thinned down to just two and I knew home was not far away. Ahead was the familiar and reassuring sight of traffic lights and queuing cars. As I continued, buildings of increasing density lined the route. Finally, I was passing through central London. It was dark and wet, but the streets were filled with light, from the cars, the windows, the lamps. The raindrops reflected the lamp light and gave the city's colours a muted beauty. I was happy to return home.

Hazel greeted me and almost immediately my phone rang. Hazel's face fell when I answered it. But I knew I had to: it was Amelia's solicitor.

'Sorry to call so late, I really wanted to hear how you got on,' she said.

'I've only just got home, Julia, and I've been thinking about this case all the way. It's quite a disturbing one.'

'How was she?'

'Traumatized. She's an interesting child, I feel great compassion for her.'

'Traumatized isn't going to help our defence – she's traumatized herself by committing homicide!'

'I'm thinking about that.'

'Look, can you get me the report by Friday?' she asked. 'We're running out of time and we've got a case conference with the barristers then.'

'Yes. But I haven't had Amelia's medical notes and I'll really need those. Something's worrying me and I think the notes will help.'

Before a GP surgery can supply notes, someone has to read them through and redact where necessary – for instance, if there are references to other people. This can be a long, slow process. Too long and too slow.

'I mean,' said Julia angrily, as if someone was arguing with her, 'what are they doing at that surgery all day?'

'Seeing patients?' I suggested.

'Oh yeah? Well, I happen to know the notes are redacted but no one's signed them off. I think that GP should put down his golf clubs and get on with his job!'

Julia was one of those people who works very hard and is convinced that, while she toils, everyone else is having fun in the sun.

She said: 'I'll have to start a major hassle offensive at the surgery.'

I doubted that any GP could easily ignore a major hassle offensive from Julia. So I approached my next question cautiously.

'Julia, there's something else I need to do.'

'Oh no, how long will this something take?'

'Do you know much about the mother's condition?'

Julia missed a beat while she thought. Characteristically, it was a very short beat. 'I gather Mrs Stickland's alive but only just. She did manage to give the police a statement, of course.'

'Is she in hospital in London?'

'No, somewhere near where they lived. Possibly Beaconsfield. Or is it Oxford?'

'Could you find out which hospital? I'd like to see her if she's able to speak.'

'Whoaa! I need that report by Friday!'

Time was tight. But I knew I must see Mrs Stickland. There was an insistence in Amelia's voice in my head. So much was missing from this jigsaw and she seemed to be telling me that her mother held the pieces.

'I think it could be very helpful to Amelia's case,' I said.

Julia agreed to find out and get back to me.

'How was it?' Hazel asked as we finally sat down together.

'Interesting.'

I tried to observe our agreement this time; that we don't discuss cases at home.

'So, what have you been doing?' I asked.

'Working on a new song, want to hear it?'

I did want to hear it. The song was lovely. We were talking about the best way for me to accompany her when I noticed the time.

'Oh! I'd better phone my mother.'

'Now? Isn't it a bit late?'

'She'll be waiting up for me.'

Did Hazel's face fall again? Or did I imagine it?

At lunchtime the next day, Amelia's notes arrived, no doubt as a result of Julia's hassle offensive. I had barely looked through them when she rang, but I had already established that, although Amelia was only twelve, her notes ran into megabytes.

They documented a complex medical history. In our interview, Amelia had referred to missing a lot of school. That was certainly true. She had caught every childhood bug possible. And she had frequently been ill, often very suddenly – in fact, she was a regular at A&E. She seemed to be plagued by a recurring infection. Generally, she spent one night in hospital on intravenous antibiotics, and then returned home.

'Are the notes useful?' Julia demanded.

'Very. Thanks for chasing them.'

'Still want to see the mother?'

'I want to see her even more now.'

'Okay. Well she's at the John Radcliffe in Oxford. I've got the number of the ward for you.'

'I'll phone them and arrange to go tomorrow if possible.'

'It will have to be tomorrow. You're finishing the report by Friday, don't forget!'

By the time I had finished reading the notes, it was time to visit my mother. I crossed London through busy traffic in the rain.

28

I found my mother in bed as usual, her small, paralysed legs hardly visible as bumps under the bedclothes. She seldom left her room now and it was like a hospital ward, with the wheelchair in one corner and bottles and boxes of medication stacked on every surface.

'I was expecting you half an hour ago!' she said as soon as she saw me. I wished my arrival made her smile. My mother was always an attractive woman. Now she was in her mid-seventies and her long struggle to get out there, to live a full life, to do what everyone else does so easily, well, now that struggle was etched on her face. Until she smiled. My mother smiling didn't just change her face, it changed the light levels, the air, every molecule in the room.

'Can you empty the commode?' she asked.

I didn't like this job but I would have to do it. The smell in here was terrible.

'That's what carers are for,' I told her as I opened the windows.

'I've only just used it and they were busy with George!' she said. 'You can't expect them to do everything – they're not here long and they knew you were coming.'

The cat was just as incontinent as my mother. Visiting them meant confronting waste in many forms. And my mother always asked me to empty the commode, even if the carers had just left. As if she'd used it when she knew

I was coming. Did it cross my mind that she enjoyed this ritual? Yes. That my revulsion in some way pleased her? Yes. I had understood years ago, when I first became a psychiatrist, that she was personality disordered. And did I love and admire her any less when I had realized that? Of course not.

I would have liked to shut my eyes, but lifting the pan and carrying it to the bathroom required their use. I felt waves of nausea. It was a relief to flush the toilet, to rinse the pan, flush again, open the bathroom window.

It was quiet outside now, and almost still, apart from the traffic which passed the front of the house. I looked out into the garden, overgrown and lit only through the bathroom window. I thought of Amelia. She came into my head at the most unexpected moments. But why now?

'Duncan! What's taking you so long in there?' my mother called.

I breathed the fresh air as it flowed in. I leaned out and noticed for the first time that ivy was growing on the outside wall, spreading upwards in tentacles like tender, outstretched hands.

'Can you see to the cat tray as well?' my mother said as I returned.

'I thought the carers had done that?'

'George has used it since!'

What was it about the interval between the carers' departure and my arrival which caused mass bowel evacuation in this house? I emptied the tray.

'You were so late that I started to worry,' my mother said as I returned once more.

I began: 'It was raining and the traffic was –'

'But why didn't you ring?'

'I warned you the traffic might be –'

'But I'd started to worry!'

I took a deep breath.

'How are you?' I asked.

'I'm worrying about my scan.'

My heart went out to her. So far as someone with polio can, she had avoided doctors all her life. Until she was diagnosed with lung cancer.

'You've a few weeks before you need to even think about it. And the scan's nothing to worry about, it's just routine,' I said.

'Can't you come with me? The consultants are different when they've got another doctor to talk to.'

'Patient Transport's booked and I'm supposed to be in court that day and you probably won't even see a doctor. I can talk to the oncologist when she's got the scan results.'

My mother sighed. 'Anyway, it will make a nice change to get out, I must say. I'm looking forward to driving myself down a sunny road in my car soon!'

I glanced out of the window. It was raining again.

I remembered the blue Motability mini my mother drove when I was a kid. It had required a lot of pushing and pulling of levers to change gear, a great flapping of elbows like bird wings. It had sometimes really felt that my mother was trying to fly when she drove it.

Design had come a long way since then and the Vauxhall was automatic. But now my mother looked too small, too frail to handle even this car and in truth it really was a long time since she had driven it.

She had only recently been told she had cancer. She was reluctant to admit that this was in any way connected to her smoking: after all, she had given up years ago.

By the time the cancer was discovered, it was disseminated through other parts of her body. But she had recently been given new medication which had been well publicized for showing remarkable results.

'I'm sure the scan results will be good,' she said. 'I'm feeling so much better with that drug. Go and start my car, will you, Duncan, to make sure the battery doesn't let me down when I need it again.'

She filled me with compassion. As usual. I did as I was told, the way I always had. Without resentment. With the same compliance I had shown as a small child asked to carry the dinner plates and hang out the washing.

When I came back in, my hair wet, I said: 'I was near Middlesbrough yesterday. And I remembered how you and Dad took me to a Chinese restaurant there once for a treat. I think I was about seven . . .'

Her eyes narrowed. For years we had hardly mentioned my father. Just hearing his name seemed to frighten her. But more recently we had occasionally talked about him, and her tone had been a little softer and we had even managed to make our family life sound normal by remembering normal things, like the Chinese restaurant.

'Oh, I think we did go and have a meal out together one day. It was lovely, a real treat,' my mother said unexpectedly.

I had been reviewing my memories of my father lately. Of course, I was still asking myself why I was so willing to forgive my mother when I had found she was the effective cause of my brain fistula – after being downright angry when I had believed it was my father's fault. It had been so easy to blame my violent father. It was easy to blame him for everything. Because there were too many spaces in my memory where the truth should be, coloured too many times by subsequent events, by my mother's stories.

I had been notified of his death and invited by his second family to see his body when I was a young doctor. It had been almost twenty years, but I approached the coffin slowly, like a child, with all the fear for my father that I had harboured as a child, bolstered by my mother's terror. I half expected him to spring from the coffin and start punching me. But when I saw his body I found that I was simply looking at another human being.

Here he was, the man I had internalized as a monster, lying helplessly. And suddenly it broke my heart that I did not know him better, that I had not made a more strenuous attempt to find him and talk to him and get to know him as something more than a monster.

I searched his face for the features I remembered, for my own features. I recalled how much I had wanted him to be my Captain Haddock, that scary, violent drunk who nevertheless loves and protects Tintin. Wondering now why Dad had neither loved nor protected me, I stared and stared. This man was inside me and always would be. But who was he?

He had married a woman who already had three daughters and to my astonishment it was clear all of them loved him deeply and mourned him greatly. At the funeral, a song he adored was played, 'Chanson d'Amour'. And then, surprisingly, came Queen.

'Queen,' his widow informed me, 'was his favourite band.'

I hadn't even known that about him.

After the funeral I was invited to his house. It was warm and neat and unpretentious and there were no signs of broken plates, no stains on the wall caused by hurled dinners, no blood on the carpet. His widow and stepdaughters regaled me with stories that made him sound like . . . well, an ordinary person. In later years he worked as a film extra and they collapsed into laughter as they told how the director had called for retakes when the extra's glasses were spotted falling off in the background. Their laughter turned to tears of grief. Could they really be talking about the same man?

One of them had a light-bulb moment.

'That box!' she cried.

I was sent upstairs to the room my father had shared with the stranger who was my stepmother. There was a dressing table covered in little bottles and some family photos. A small one at the back featured a thin boy looking crushed inside the arm of a young man: the man was younger than I was now. His hair was seventies wild; there was a big moustache, a winning smile. I remembered that boy, that man. Had they stood on the dressing table all these years in this still, silent room?

The box was where they had said it would be. It was a shoe box. Leather uppers, size ten.

Inside was a school photo, unframed, a boy squinting shyly into the camera. I unfolded a small piece of paper and found a picture. Drawn by a child and drawn with care. I had been sitting on the floor at my uncle's waiting for the adults to finish talking, and my uncle had given me a pen and paper, I remembered that.

And here was a tiny hospital wrist band. Handwritten on it was Baby Harding, Male. And my date of birth.

There was a small plastic toy, something I might have prized once but which was now long forgotten. Another school picture, tiny this time. In it I was missing a front tooth. A neatly folded poster for the gig at the Working Men's Club, when I had last seen him. And, finally, a printed-out copy of my General Medical Council registration. So he had known that I was a doctor and evidently he was proud of it.

The box shouted to me of an extraordinary possibility. That my father had loved me.

I felt the axis of my world shift. This man, who had seldom entered my thoughts for years but was somehow always there, had loved me. I sat down on the edge of the bed that he shared with his second wife and felt hot tears fall. This possibility, of love, was one I had never considered.

'But what does that change, really?' I asked myself when I had said goodbye to my mother and George the cat and was driving home through London's traffic, still remembering my father's funeral. I didn't know. But I knew it changed something.

When I arrived home, Hazel was going to bed.

'We had to fill in some forms for social services,' I explained. 'You know what she's like, she argues about every word.'

Hazel smiled patiently. She knew that, whenever I visited my mother, there were always some forms to fill in, things to fix, change, amend, organize. Something to detain me.

My phone rang. It was my mother. Hazel looked at me quizzically.

'Duncan!' My mother never bothered with any of the usual phone greetings. 'Are you back yet? You didn't call me and you know how I worry!'

'I just walked in . . .'

Her voice softened. 'I wanted to say that it was very nice to see you. But I thought to myself: he's looking tired. I hope you're not working too hard, that wife of yours should tell you to rest.'

Hazel was a busy doctor too. She needed to rest just as much as I did, but my mother did not prioritize her. On our wedding day, I had arranged a disabled taxi for my mother but she had arrived at the wedding in a wheelchair, feeling slighted because I had not picked her up personally. Her sadness did affect me, but it could not prevent our wedding day from being one of the happiest of my life.

'I'm going to rest right now,' I assured her.

When I shut my eyes in bed that night, I dreamed of my father. We were driving past mile after mile of lamps towards some distant and unnamed destination. And, in my dream, the middle-aged man behind the wheel and the young boy driven into the darkness with his father were the same person.

29

Ten o'clock the next morning found me at the John Radcliffe to visit Amelia's mother. One of the many consultants I'd worked with had transferred here and set up a famous clinic: the old-school Tourette's specialist. I recalled his tweedy jackets. His shooting ties. And how he carried a sense of hierarchy and maintained a distant froideur with both junior doctors and patients. Once he had dropped a book off in my office.

'Oh, thanks, mate,' I'd said, unthinkingly.

From the doorway, he swung around to face me.

'You do not,' he said, 'call me mate.'

'Oh. Sorry.'

'And, while we're on the subject, I've seen you call patients mate as well. Duncan, that is entirely, *entirely*, inappropriate.'

Occasionally calling patients mate or discussing Harry Potter if they happened to be fans, or *Dr Who* or *Wipeout* or trains or music or anything we shared an interest in, well, that was how I made patients feel relaxed and hopefully helped them to talk with me. This approach was the opposite of that old-style consultant's methods. He would no more have shared an interest with a patient than with a door handle. He thought I called people mate because of my working-class background. He didn't know that the tide was going out on his style of medicine, which relied on an assumption of the doctor's superiority.

But people are so complex. Because despite all that, he was fundamentally a nice man and we got on well and he generously taught me a lot. He had retired now but, if he had still been working here, I would certainly have dropped in to see him before finding Amelia's mother.

I arrived on Mrs Stickland's ward and, although I hadn't planned to, some instinct suddenly made me ask for a nurse to sit in on the interview. I felt that I might need to follow the strictest of protocols with Amelia's mother.

The room was alongside the ward. The nurse bustled in, explaining that Mrs Stickland was being treated for third degree burns. I introduced myself to the figure in the bed, who seemed to be bandaged from head to foot. Even her face was bandaged, except for her eyes and mouth. Her eyes were shut. She neither moved nor spoke. I felt discouraged. As if someone had slammed a door in my face.

I completed my introduction but she said nothing. I could see she was not asleep. So I waited for her. The nurse and I exchanged glances and I shrugged. Minutes passed. I continued to wait.

Mrs Stickland had survived the fire by jumping from a first-floor window. Her husband had rushed to save Jay-Jay, and neither of them had made it out of the house. According to the fire chief's report, the flames would have flashed through in an instant, fuelled by all the petrol. In fact, he was amazed that Mrs Stickland had managed to save herself. And now, her only family member left in the world was the daughter who had started the fatal fire. Here was certainly a woman suffering from extreme shock and grief. Of course, she had slammed the door on me. Let her take her time before opening it.

Maybe she was expecting me to say something. But I wouldn't do that. I wasn't here to listen to my own voice. So the painful silence continued.

Finally, after about eight awkward minutes, during which the nurse, clearly anxious to return to her duties, shuffled quite a lot, Mrs Stickland's eyes opened.

'Yes?' she said.

I had positioned myself, not directly in front of her but where she could see me if she chose to. Although, she didn't choose to. She looked instead at the ceiling. And she said: 'Yes?' in exactly the tone used by that tweedy consultant I had worked with, as if I was someone very junior who was wasting the time of a busy and important person.

Careful, Duncan. I recognized that the thoughts I'd had about this case made me predisposed to disliking Mrs Stickland. I should certainly put aside all such feelings. I looked for, and found, some compassion inside me for the woman who lay suffering helplessly in the hospital bed. But I acknowledged to myself how strange it was that, despite Mrs Stickland's terrible trauma, I had caught myself sympathizing with the fire's perpetrator rather than its victim.

I said: 'Thanks for speaking to me, Mrs Stickland. I met Amelia yesterday.'

I paused. I didn't expect her to say anything to that, and she didn't.

'I'm writing a report about the fire, from a psychiatric perspective.'

Still nothing. 'I'm very sorry, I know this must be

extremely difficult for you and I really do appreciate your agreeing to see me.'

Silence. She wasn't going to make things easier. I wondered if she was enjoying my discomfort, then banished the thought.

'The court case is actually scheduled for next month,' I said. 'The evidence that Amelia started the fire is strong. I have read your police interview but I'm left with a few more questions of my own. I'd like to talk to you about Amelia, about what happened that day. I'm wondering if you can make sense of any of it.'

She did not speak. Her eyes blinked.

Suddenly the awfulness of her journey hit me. How the busy mother of two had become this silent, motionless, bandaged patient.

'It must all feel . . . impossible,' I said.

A weak attempt at acknowledging Mrs Stickland's pain. But it was enough, because now she spoke.

'Not really.' She lifted a bandaged arm. 'It was possible.' The arm gave something like a wave. Then she dropped it. 'Very possible.'

She was talking at last and I didn't want her to stop, so I rapidly asked another question. Something innocuous about the day of the fire, what she had done, how the weather had been.

Silence.

So that was a mistake. After a minute or two, I decided to go straight to the heart of the matter. I had nothing to lose.

I said: 'After the fire, Forensics examined what was left, of course . . .'

She gave something like a snort and the snort said that there was nothing left. Of her house, of her life.

'. . . and they found something in your bedroom that they didn't really understand. In a drawer.'

Fire is a strange marauder. It freakishly leaves areas, objects, crannies, whole shelves untouched, while ravaging everything else nearby.

'They found a small bag. And inside it were syringes. Well, Forensics thought that's what they were.'

I watched her closely but saw no response.

'I was wondering why you had syringes in your room?'

I hoped that was the right tone. It seemed unlikely that she was a drug addict, but if she was, then I didn't want her to feel judged.

She looked directly at me now. Her eyes were open but they were blank. Completely blank, as if she had died in the fire. I persisted.

'Amelia mentioned in passing that she had missed a lot of school. I was curious to know why. In her medical notes, I saw that she was often admitted to A&E, always with the same infection.'

She continued to stare at me. She did not speak. She did not swallow. She did not move at all. I already had my suspicions about the sort of thing the syringes might have contained and I had contacted the lab. They had simply been listed on a forensic report along with other personal items which had survived the fire. No one had actually analysed them. I had asked the lab to do so and was now awaiting their results.

Mrs Stickland said nothing. Finally, I broke the long silence.

'I believe,' I said, 'that you've been seeing your own psychiatrist for quite some time.' The psychiatrist's invoices had been listed on the inventory of things saved from the fire. 'Could you tell me anything about that?'

'Why?'

I realized that I had mistaken the tone in her voice earlier. I had thought her haughty and dismissive. On the way here, I had been remembering a doctor at this very hospital who could be haughty and dismissive and now I had misinterpreted Mrs Stickland's tone as the same. I really should be more careful, I thought. I strive to keep interviews unfiltered by my own story, by my preconceptions, by ideas I might be forming around a case. But no one can do that entirely successfully, or not without a lot of careful self-scrutiny. Now I admitted to myself that Mrs Stickland's tone wasn't arrogant. It was flat. Death in her eyes, death in her voice.

I said: 'I'm looking for ways to help.'

No movement, no sound.

'I'd like to speak to your psychiatrist. If you'd agree? I'd just need a signature.'

'Why?' Her voice was croaky but there was force in it. 'Why, why, why? I didn't start the fucking fire. Ask Amelia.'

The nurse had stopped fidgeting some minutes ago and now she was absolutely motionless. As the room grew darker, we both stared at the ghostly figure of Mrs Stickland, sitting among the white sheets, shrouded in white bandages. When we had first entered, slanted sunlight had lain across one end of the bed. Now the sun had moved and its light no longer fell between the buildings. There was a new coolness in the air.

I said: 'It's helpful for me to get a picture of your family life. So some idea of your diagnosis would be very useful. Are you aware of any diagnosis?'

Of course, she didn't answer. But in the end, perhaps just to get rid of me, she gave me permission to contact her psychiatrist. I knew that was the most I could hope for from her. I thanked her and wished her well, not expecting a response, not getting one. As I left the ward, I felt relief. Stepping outside, the fresh air felt just as welcoming as the air on the right side of prison gates.

As Amelia's trial grew closer, I could hardly sleep. I had submitted my report and attended a case conference. The trial was still a few weeks away, but I could not stop thinking about her case. Amelia was inside my head: her patterns of speech, her voice, her cadences. If I fell asleep, I woke abruptly and each time from a dream in which Amelia was trying to tell me something. It was something she'd been telling me all along but I hadn't been listening.

London's heart never stops beating and even in the depth of the night I could hear the great city moving outside. Drunks arguing. Distant sirens. A motorbike, its roar cutting through the dull thrum of car engines and the chugging of night boats on their journeys down the river towards the sea. The Thames keeps on flowing.

I listened to it all, night after night, hour after hour, envying Hazel her deep sleep. What, I kept asking myself, was Amelia trying to tell me? I thought of her small face, her constant scab-picking. I remembered the way she pushed and pulled and even chewed at certain places on her arm. Did she create small wounds in the first place through self-harm which had turned into scabs? I had asked her carer about self-harm and she had shaken her head. There was no mention of it in any medical notes. Perhaps an allergy had caused the problem, but there was no doubt that she was making it much worse by constantly worrying at it.

Then something occurred to me, a thought that was so sudden and powerful it was like an electrical charge. I sat up in bed. Consciously or unconsciously, had Amelia been drawing attention to the scabs themselves?

By morning, I had a theory. I was picking and pulling at it, the way Amelia had picked and pulled at the scabs. Hazel left for work as I made a coffee and went straight back to the bundle to re-read it. All of it. I had already sent Mrs Stickland's psychiatrist a scan of the permission she had signed but so far I had not succeeded in talking to him. Now I dialled his number once more. And this time he answered.

He confirmed that Mrs Stickland had been referred to him by her GP suffering from acute anxiety some years ago. He had continued to see her privately. He talked about the anxiety, about mixed personality issues. That was no surprise. Depression. No surprises there either. No psychosis, no bipolar affective disorder . . .

I arranged to return to the John Radcliffe the following day. I wanted to discuss my theory with Mrs Stickland – not that I expected her to join in the discussion. And there she was, in the same bed, in the same room, off the same ward. Although a different nurse sat with us this time.

A few bandages had been removed from her face and I could see her features more clearly now. How could I ever have thought her haughty? The bandages had simply exposed further suffering. She really was a ghost. I tried to look past the tragic victim to the woman Amelia had known before: demanding, difficult and disordered.

She stared at me vacantly and said little. But she said enough. I contacted Julia and told her that I wanted to provide an addendum report.

30

As usual, I was nervous before my court appearance. I would be discussing Amelia with a barrister I had found to be formidable at case conference. I just hoped that the prosecution barrister wasn't nearly as formidable. It would be my job, more than any other witness, to explain to the jury that Amelia's mental health condition meant that she had not been capable of forming intent to kill, and that her condition substantially affected her decision-making ability on the day of the fire. If we were successful, she would not go to jail but to hospital where, in my view, she belonged.

Amelia sat in the dock looking ridiculously small, like a tiny bird in a big cage. Her age meant that this case was entirely below the media's radar. The public seats were empty. The press benches were empty too. Apart from officials and those of us working directly on the case, the courtroom was a strange, quiet void.

Amelia's intermediary, a middle-aged woman, sat close to her behind the Perspex screen, whispering sometimes: it was her job to recognize if Amelia needed a break and to make sure she understood all that happened.

I did look at Amelia for a moment as I took the affirmation. She gazed back at me. Her face was empty. As empty as her mother's stare. I gave her a quick half-smile. Her expression did not change.

By now I had gained much more experience as an expert witness and the bungling of my earlier years on the stand was seldom repeated – although I lived in fear of it.

I stood in the witness box; I had learned never to sit down but to stand respectfully and remember always to whom I was talking. The jury, of course. But it is very tempting to answer questions by turning to face the barrister who asks them, especially in such an empty courtroom.

I knew it was going to be a long afternoon. I rocked backwards and forwards on my feet to promote blood flow and give me stamina while I waited for the first question.

It was an easy one, of course, from our barrister. Here was a chance to state my qualifications, experience and expertise clearly and, without false modesty, to show the jury why they had to take my conclusions seriously.

Mr Piantono, our defence barrister, escorted me through the report I'd written. From the outset, every question was designed for me to give the answer we wanted. It was like being handed a piece of cake and told to eat it. Knowing all the time that the prosecution would cross-examine me next and all they wanted me to eat was humble pie.

We recalled details of the fire, of Amelia, as we worked our way slowly towards the nub of my evidence.

'Amelia killed two people and maimed one, nobody in this room is disputing that. Do you believe, Dr Harding, it was her intention to kill her family? That she set fire to the house because she wanted them to die?'

I paused.

'I think that Amelia intended, at some level, to burn the

house down. But this is a very complex case. And there are various factors which affected her capacity to form an intent to kill that night.'

'Could you tell the jury the most important of those factors, please?'

'I believe that Amelia was suffering from severe complex trauma, resulting in post-traumatic stress disorder. This complex trauma has many symptoms, the most relevant being a detached state of mind at times of extreme stress. In my opinion, her traumatized state reduced her capacity to form intent.'

Mr Piantono nodded and looked very serious.

'Now Amelia was, up until this incident, a normal schoolgirl with average grades. Why do you believe that she was actually suffering from a traumatic disorder?'

'At home, nothing was normal. In my opinion, she suffered from trauma inflicted by her mother over a number of years.'

'What form did the trauma take?'

'I believe that Amelia's mother has Munchausen syndrome by proxy. That is best explained by describing Munchausen syndrome. Sufferers are driven by a need to experience the care and sympathy of others. They are usually completely unconscious of this need but, in order to meet it, they invent a physical illness and present their symptoms to doctors, to hospitals.'

'Now you are not claiming that anyone in this case suffers from Munchausen syndrome, is that right?'

'I am not. I –'

The prosecution barrister was on his feet appealing to the judge like a footballer feigning injury to the referee.

'Your honour, why do we have to hear about some irrelevant disorder? No one suffers from this syndrome, by Dr Harding's own admission! He is simply confusing the jury!'

But try as the prosecution might to prevent me, I was determined to make my point.

'I am trying to explain that I believe Amelia's mother has Munchausen syndrome *by proxy*.'

The prosecution barrister looked pained. 'Your honour, we are not here to discuss Amelia's mother and syndromes she may or may not have!'

Mr Piantono jumped in.

'Your honour, I assure you this has the utmost relevance to the defence's case.'

The judge paused to consider. Finally, she nodded. 'Very well, Mr Piantono, Dr Harding may continue.'

There was a pause from Mr Piantono in which he seemed to regain control of the room. The best barristers know how to weaponize silence.

He looked at the jury. 'So we have learned that patients with Munchausen syndrome visit doctors or admit themselves to hospital when there is nothing wrong with them . . .' He turned to me. 'So what, then, is Munchausen syndrome by proxy?'

'A patient with Munchausen by proxy shows the same unconscious needs as someone with Munchausen syndrome. But this time, the patient is untruthful about a physical illness that affects *another* person. That other person is a proxy vessel for illness. Sometimes the vessel is their own child. The child is taken to the doctor or the hospital when there is nothing wrong. Sometimes, the child is actually made ill, I mean, harmed, for the Munchausen sufferer – usually the parent – to receive the attention they crave.'

'And on what do you base your evidence that Mrs Stickland has Munchausen by proxy?'

'I have spoken to her psychiatrist and he said it was a strong possibility. I first began to realize that this might be the case when syringes were found in Mrs Stickland's room. They seemed strange but not significant. Until I saw Amelia's arms. When she was first arrested, the duty doctor's report notes the multiple puncture marks on her arms and her thighs – they were similar to the track marks we might find on the body of a heroin addict.'

I didn't say that Amelia had picked at them, turned them into scabs, picked at them again and continued to pick at them, enlarging and exaggerating them over time. Until the scabs were shouting, not whispering. I did not confess how long it had taken me to hear them.

The jury sat very still. None of them wrote notes or looked as if they would rather be phoning a friend. They all stared directly at me.

'So,' said Mr Piantono gently, 'syringes were found and there was evidence of injections on the arms of the accused. So you are suggesting that Mrs Stickland used the syringes to inject something into her daughter that made her ill?'

'There is further evidence for this in Amelia's medical notes. Amelia was very frequently admitted to A&E over a number of years, each time with a severe but not life-threatening infection. Far more frequently than one would expect in an otherwise healthy child. So I believe that Mrs

Stickland was harming her daughter and Amelia knew that. This knowledge caused Amelia's complex traumatic state. I don't think she was able to compute what the consequences of her action might be on the night she started the fire. I think she was so traumatized that she was incapable of forming the intention to kill.'

Every so often, when a courtroom goes very quiet and still, when every face looks thoughtful or withdrawn, when the jury seems frozen in their seats, you can be fairly sure that the verdict will go the way you believe it should.

Except that the prosecution barrister was not going to give in without a fight.

When it was his turn to cross-examine me, he leaned towards me like a man leaning on the bar at the pub. Barristers can be at their most dangerous when they look matey.

'Evidence, Dr Harding! I believe, I think, it is my opinion . . . we have heard those words very often from you, but you have no real *evidence* for your theory. Let's look at the facts, not a series of conjectures. You have already admitted to them. You agree that the defendant preplanned the murder of her family. In fact, you have listed the ways in which she planned it – and planned *with purpose*. Your report says that the petrol was laid in the house in advance, you agree that she had stowed cash in a secret place in order to make her getaway on the night of the fire. Nothing in your report suggests that these murders occurred in a moment of madness. That's correct, isn't it?'

No point arguing. I said: 'Yes, it's correct.'

'Yes,' he repeated. 'Yes!' His voice was booming now. We'd left the pub and seemed to have stumbled into the pulpit. 'Those are the facts and yet you have chosen to replace them with some wild theory of your own. Let's go through that theory. First, you claim that Mrs Stickland suffers from something called Munchausen syndrome by proxy which caused her to make her daughter ill. But, as I understand it, even her own psychiatrist could not confirm this.'

'He knows his patient well enough to recognize the possibility. He had no evidence to confirm it.'

'That is because there is no evidence, Dr Harding. A syringe found here, marks on a girl's arm there – nothing, nothing connects the two beyond a rather extravagant hypothesis. And, according to that same hypothesis, a mother injecting her child with some foreign matter is enough for you to relieve the child of responsibility for the two deaths she has caused. Would you please be kind enough to tell the court how you consider that to be the case?'

Here was scorn masquerading as manners. But I was determined not to falter.

'Our parents should love us and protect us and care for us. They should keep us safe. That is the least children have a right to expect. When a parent withdraws protection and harms a child in such a calculated way over a long period, the consequences for the child are severe, because the harm caused by this knowledge may well exceed the physical harm inflicted. Amelia suffered the drip, drip of chronic abuse over years. She lived in a state of extreme emotional overwhelm. I believe that this resulted in a detached state of mind. Perhaps she fantasized about setting fire to the house, but that in my view is not the same as enactment. The best diagnostic fit for this level of detachment, a level which undermined her ability to make decisions or form intent to kill, would be complex trauma resulting in post-traumatic stress disorder.'

I did not look at Amelia but I knew she was looking at me. While the jury's eyes slid from me to Amelia then back.

Only the prosecution barrister maintained a sceptical expression.

'You have no proof for your theory! You have not even suggested what might have been in those alleged syringes.'

I shifted uncomfortably from foot to foot. I knew exactly what was in the syringes because Forensics had finally informed me that very morning. There had been no time to tell the defence team and I knew it wasn't right to throw a new piece of evidence into the case at this stage.

I said: 'Your honour, I would like to discuss my evidence with Mr Piantoni, if I may be given five minutes.'

The prosecution barrister objected to this most strongly. The judge agreed with him.

'If you have evidence, please just give it in open court, Dr Harding,' she instructed.

I glanced apologetically at our defence counsel and took a deep breath.

'The syringes contained human faeces.'

Silence: guaranteed. Movement in the room: non-existent. Coughing, sneezing, shuffling: zero.

I had returned to Mrs Stickland's bedside in Oxford and told her my theory, but I really had not expected her to say anything. I was amazed when she had spoken. Just to say that one word: 'Yes.' Before closing her eyes and shutting me out.

When I glanced at the jury's faces and saw their compassion for Amelia, I was sure of our verdict. They returned within an hour. This was not murder, as the prosecution had proposed, but manslaughter with diminished responsibility. Amelia would not be sent to a children's jail but to a psychiatric hospital where she would be given help, support and treatment.

I did see her afterwards, in that place she was being held, somewhere in the labyrinth under the court. Julia was outside Amelia's cell. She was less brisk than usual.

'Thanks, Duncan. Good work. So! Hey! We won.'

'It doesn't feel like there are any winners,' I said.

Julia nodded agreement.

Amelia's head was bowed and she sat very still. Too still. I wished she would pick her scabs. She was wearing a voluminous but childish dress which covered them up, covered her whole body.

'Do you want to talk?' I asked.

She stared at the ground. She shook her head.

I said: 'Good luck, Amelia.'

I turned as I was leaving the room and for a moment she looked up and her eyes met mine. I smiled at her. I did not expect her to smile back.

Outside the court, the streets were busy, the people were busy, all London was busy. It would have been good to walk busily away from the case now it was over. I would almost certainly not encounter Amelia again. But it wasn't so easy to leave her behind.

At the tube station, I began my descent beneath the city, jostled by office workers and tourists.

My phone buzzed in my pocket.

'Dr Harding, it's Parminder Sharp, do you remember me?'

'Hi Parminder, of course I do. You're Layla's solicitor. How is she, do you know?'

'In a bit of trouble.'

'Oh no!'

'I remember this was a case you felt very strongly about . . . I'm wondering if you can help us out.'

Layla was in trouble. The news both surprised and distressed me.

'Is now the right time to discuss it? Sounds like you're in a busy place.'

'Getting on the tube, so we'll be cut off any minute, I'll call you as soon as I'm home.'

'No, I'm still liaising with the police on this; just wanted to check that you're up for it. I'll get back to you soon.'

The tube thundered into the dark tunnel and I wished she had told me what sort of trouble Layla could be in. The occasional reappearance of an offender, especially someone I have defended in the past, always gives me a sinking feeling. It invariably means recidivism and usually indicates that I made a mistake, perhaps by assessing a defendant's risk poorly. That we make occasional mistakes is something we have to accept or we wouldn't sleep at night. But Layla? Layla of all people? Inside my head, Amelia shrank just a little bit, to make room for her.

31

My mother's scan results were, as she had predicted, encouraging. The tumour in her lungs had shrunk by half in just three months.

'I'll be back in my car again soon!' she said excitedly.

I looked at the oncologist. She spent so much of her life giving people bad news. Now she had made someone happy. Of course, she was smiling back at my mother.

'You've kept the car battery charged, haven't you, Duncan?' my mother asked.

I nodded as she spun off to tell the nurses the good news.

Her reaction was scarcely credible to me. I had lived with my mother's threats of suicide throughout my childhood; in fact, the constant, low-level worry that she would end her life didn't really start to lift until I was in my thirties. But when the oncologist had asked if she really wanted to prolong life with unpleasant and highly aggressive chemotherapy, she had answered, without hesitation: 'Yes, oh yes!'

Then she was offered a new medication and she had agreed at once. I could not believe that she was fighting so hard for life when she had previously treated it like something old and cheap that she was always on the verge of discarding.

I was left in the room with the oncologist. Her smile faded.

'So . . . how long has she got?' I asked quietly.

'Literally, no idea. This drug is a big unknown. That sort of tumour shrinkage is in excess of its usual results.'

I felt my heart miss a beat with excitement. Could my frail mother really be driving her car again soon? Even though I knew this was irrational, I allowed myself to feel hope.

'So if the cancer keeps on shrinking at the same rate . . .'

The oncologist raised her eyebrows. 'We just don't know. The results look good now, but of course this drug isn't curative.'

Oh, this instinct, of my mother's, of mine, of the doctors', of almost everyone, to prolong life. Even though her life had become so limited and low in quality. She loved me, and her old cat, but she was now dependent on carers in a way that she once would have hated. And her world was getting smaller. She had been an avid reader since childhood, but now she spent her days watching reruns of *Flog It!*

I must have been thinking out loud, because the oncologist said:

'It may not be your idea of quality of life but it's enough for Mrs Harding.'

I nodded humbly. I said: 'I'm writing a book and . . . I'd like her to live to see it published.'

She pulled a face.

'Don't know how quickly you write, but certainly it will need to be in print within the next two years. I mean, really, this drug is full of surprises. She might have two years, but she might only have three months.'

I heard two years. To three months, I chose deafness. It

is a necessary part of life's natural cycle for parents to die, but I could not contemplate my mother's absence. Not imagine my life without focusing daily on her needs and health, as I had all my life. It would be like living next to a mountain and finding it gone one day.

Later I sat at my desk, watched as usual by Dr Who and Tintin. Work had piled up and my phone did not stop ringing.

'Hey Duncan, it's Will. Remember Callum?'

Ah Callum. That early forensic case, the boy who had been rude and hostile and had called me a spaz and a dickhead throughout the interview. Had I really agreed that some ADHD medication might sort him out? Since then, I had learned a thing or two. I had learned that amphetamine salts did not work so well behind bars as behind the school door. And I had sometimes wondered if Callum would come bouncing back.

'Things are looking a bit grim,' said Will. 'Could you see him again?'

'What's happened? Did he take his ADHD medication?'

'No. He wouldn't take it. Refused to engage with health services. Told them all to fuck off, I believe.'

My heart sank.

'Oh. So . . . what's he done now?'

'He's attacked and hospitalized two boys. One of them has broken bones. The other one was shot.'

'Shot! Callum had a gun?'

Callum and a gun was an unthinkable combination.

'Yeah,' said Will gloomily. 'Of course he won't say where he got it.'

'What happened?'

'You can see for yourself on the CCTV footage if you've got the stomach for it.'

'I mean, what happened to the victim?'

'Callum shot towards the boy's abdomen – rather inexpertly, in my opinion. I think it was the first time he'd used the gun. Anyway, the bullet went through his body without touching any major organs or blood vessels. Lucky lad.'

'Unlucky lad,' I said, 'to find himself within range of Callum's gun.'

'It looks like a bit of revenge. These two attacked one of Callum's mates so Callum felt honour-bound to get them. That's a direct quote. Honour-bound. For God's sake.'

'So it was a gang thing?'

'I think so. Callum started off by throwing one of the boys around. Bruises plus a few bones broken. Then the other lad had a go and Callum simply reached for his gun and shot him.'

'Does he show any remorse?'

'No. He believes he did the right thing because these two attacked his mate.'

I groaned.

'It was gang warfare,' Will said dramatically, 'so we can't assume that Callum was the ringleader.'

I tried not to assume that, but it was hard.

'Do you have witness statements?'

'Yes, along with the CCTV. Shall I send the whole bundle over?'

'Okay, and do you want me to interview him again?'

'Worth a try, he might be more helpful this time. The thing is . . . it's really urgent. Could you interview him and get the report done this week?'

I sighed. 'I can't do it tomorrow, I'm away all day. I could interview him early on Thursday morning and get at least a preliminary report off to you then?'

'Done. Thanks, Duncan.'

Before I had finished the call, a text had arrived from Parminder Sharp about that other bounce-back case. Layla.

You know how time has rules of its own and it seems like there's lots of it and then suddenly there isn't and everything's urgent? I looked at Dr Who and nodded agreement. Yep, time has rules of its own, we both knew that. *Could you possibly get here this week to see Layla? Please?*

I messaged back that I was fully booked to interview other children and that their reports were urgent. But that I could meet Layla late on Thursday. Knowing that I did not really have time. Knowing that if Layla needed me, I must see her.

32

The very first time I met Layla, I was astonished by her. Even though I had been working hard at the NHS forensic hub for a few years and had encountered a wide variety of unusual cases, she still astonished me.

First, she was not at all what I was expecting. Despite all my intentions not to pre-form opinions, I sometimes do. Sexual offences are carried out by very young children more often than you might think, usually but not always because they have themselves been abused. But Layla had been arrested for procuring and distributing pornographic images, a charge which usually requires at least an adolescent interest in sex. I have known twelve-year-old boys who are hulking adolescents on the cusp of manhood and I have known twelve-year-old girls who present with sexual maturity. Without really examining that expectation, I walked into the secure children's unit harbouring it.

What a surprise. Layla looked about ten – or anyway, pre-pubescent.

She was polite, friendly and had a very likeable charm. This was a rare find in a secure home. It was even rarer to meet a child who seemed perfectly happy to be here.

I went through the usual questions with her and found her answers surprising.

She sat on the edge of her chair, eyes shining, alert,

ready to be helpful. She had short hair and wore a T-shirt with a picture of a horse on it. Not My Little Pony, but a photo of a real horse.

'Do you know why I'm seeing you today, Layla?'

'Yes. For court.'

'What will I do in court?'

'You will help Miss Sharp. I'm glad you're helping her, I think she's very nice, don't you?'

I nodded.

'And beautiful,' she continued. 'Miss Sharp is like a really sleek Dartmoor pony.'

Layla's voice was high. Her features had the roundness and her body the slimness of childhood. She sat up straight. Some children in her situation hunch in their chairs, reluctant to look up. Layla was the very opposite. It crossed my mind that maybe the children's unit had introduced me to the wrong patient and this was someone else whose name was Layla.

'You like ponies?'

'I love them!'

What was it about girls and ponies? I remembered how Amelia, when I had visited her in that faraway rural unit, had liked a pony. I could even remember its name. Monty.

'So, Layla, do you understand why you're staying in the unit?'

She nodded vigorously.

'Oh yes, yes I do. Because of the computer stuff.'

'So when did you move here?'

'Three weeks and four days ago.'

'Exactly three weeks and four days?'

'I could work out how many hours if you want me to!'

'No, you've been accurate enough. Have you had any visitors?'

'My family. They come every weekend and we speak on Wednesday at seven p.m.'

'And you know that I'm here to write a report on you, and some of my report will be read out in court? So it's not like going to see your doctor and –'

'Dr Ibrahim,' supplied Layla helpfully. 'He's my doctor at home.'

'Well, Dr Ibrahim won't tell anyone what you say when you go into his surgery but, even though I'm a doctor too, I will be telling people what you've said to me. All the people in court might hear it. I want to make sure you understand that.'

I noticed that I was talking to her as though she were a young child, not a nearly-thirteen-year-old.

She nodded vigorously.

'So it's okay for me to carry on? Will you sign a piece of paper saying that it's okay?'

'Oh, yes!'

Layla was helpful and signed with a smile. I had never really encountered a defendant like this, certainly not one facing such horrible charges. Pornography offenders can find it very hard to look me in the eye. Not Layla.

'Can you tell me what happened?' I began.

She seemed genuinely surprised by this question.

'But, don't you already know?'

'Miss Sharp did explain it to me, but I'd like to hear it from you. If that's okay? I hope it won't upset you too much to tell me.'

She nodded. 'So. There was a link on this chatroom I use . . .'

She named a site for children and I asked her to explain how it worked.

'You can go there and chat about the things you like. I like ponies. So, you put your topic in the box and other people who like ponies can message you.'

'What did you put in the box?'

'Well not my name, obviously. I know how to stay safe online. So just my username and what I'm specifically interested in. You could put Ponies. But then you'd get loads of messages. It's better to be more specific. Do you like ponies?'

The default position when a patient asks you a personal question is not to share, but if a child makes some innocuous enquiry, fending it off can feel brusque and unkind. I answered now, and I should say that this would be regarded by my colleagues as very poor boundary-keeping.

'I do like ponies, I like all animals really. But we're not here to talk about me today. Will you tell me what happened?'

'So, I typed: New Forest palomino. I really love many different kinds of ponies – I expect you know, if you like ponies, that there are fifteen native breeds in the British Isles. Nine of them are English and Dartmoor's my favourite but New Forest are soooo cute too. Anyway, palomino is a colour, not a breed. There's a palomino pony at the stables I visit called Sparkler and she's such a lovely gold, with a silver tail . . .'

'Do you ride Sparkler?' I asked.

'Well, Mum can't afford riding very often so I just visit.

And I'm still on the leading rein, I'm not experienced enough to ride Sparkler, but I'm allowed to brush her.'

Amelia had liked to brush Monty too. Girls and ponies didn't seem to be about riding them.

'So you typed in palomino?'

'Yes. And at first, nothing happened. That's very surprising as a lot of people like palominos. Anyway, I kept checking. Nothing! For at least a week. Then one afternoon I got home from school and there was just one message. It was from Sadie3245. She's like me, she loves ponies and she's got two! One's part-New Forest . . . and it's a palomino, I couldn't believe it! I was typing her a message asking for a picture of her pony when she sent me a link. Of course I clicked on it.'

She paused.

'Because you thought she was sending pictures of her pony?'

'Yes, I couldn't wait to see it. And these files downloaded directly into my Dropbox. I mean, automatically. I hadn't set that up, I think maybe it's a default. Anyway, I didn't mind.'

'So you clicked on the files?'

'Yes, and they all unzipped. And . . .'

I waited.

'And, there were lots of pictures. Not pictures of ponies. But . . .' She was quieter now. Her shoulders drooped a little. '. . . weird stuff. I mean, stuff with dogs and ladies and lots of the pictures had little kids. I couldn't understand it. I . . .'

She stopped speaking. Not because she was emotionally overwhelmed, it seemed to me, but because she felt confused remembering her confusion.

'What did you do, Layla?'

'Well, I wrote back to Sadie, of course, telling her she'd sent me the wrong files and I was looking forward to seeing pictures of her palomino.'

'Did she reply?'

'No.'

'These files were sexual in nature? Pornographic?'

Layla nodded sadly.

'Did you tell anyone about them?'

'No. I should have told my mum. But I didn't and I don't know why.'

'Did you look at the files?'

And for the first time, Layla could not meet my eye. She looked down, ashamed.

She said: 'I watched them. All of them.'

'How did that make you feel?'

'Sort of . . . strange. I mean, a bit sick. At first. But curious too. I . . . I couldn't stop looking at them. I looked at some of them over and over again, like I do with pony videos.'

'Did this feel different from watching ponies?'

She nodded. She still did not look at me.

'I'm sorry to ask this, Layla, I really am. Did you feel excited when you watched those things? I mean, sexually excited?'

She shook her head. Not with her previous vigour; it was just an indication of a headshake. 'Not really. I get excited when I look at ponies, especially if they're cantering. Cantering in a group is nice. But I don't feel . . . you know. Sexually excited. I'm not really into boys and stuff like that.'

'So . . . why did you watch the videos so often?'

She shook her head in confusion.

'I don't know.'

'What happened after that?'

'Well, Sadie3245 sort of replied the next day. She sent me another link. This time she didn't tell me anything about her ponies. So . . . it was there when I got back from school and I clicked on it and it downloaded a zip file and it was all just like before. Although the videos were different.'

'When you clicked on it, did you think it might be ponies?'

'Yes, I thought, aha, she's sent me the palomino this time. But I also thought: maybe she's sent me more stuff like before. So, I was sort of hoping that it was ponies and sort of hoping that it was more . . . more of that stuff. And it was. More stuff. Only different. I had to watch it. Over and over. I couldn't stop.'

'Did she send you any more links?'

'She sent one every day, day after day, well, four days in all. There were loads and loads of videos, all in my Dropbox. So, I categorized them. I prefer things to be categorized, otherwise they're just a muddle.'

'How did you categorize them?'

'It was quite hard sometimes. For instance, I had a dog folder. That was easy. And inside that folder, I had subcategories. So there was dog with lady tied up, dog with lady not tied up . . . With the kids, I did it mainly by age and that was hard because the file names didn't give ages but, anyway, I'm quite good at judging age, I think. So I had a category Age five to ten and a category Age ten to fifteen, and each of the Age categories were divided into boys and girls . . .'

Her voice faded away.

'The videos sound like quite serious stuff, Layla. Did you realize that?'

'Yes,' she said, looking down again. 'I know. I'm a paedophile.'

This was a surprising word for her to use.

'I'm a paedophile because I was looking at kids. And then there were dogs and there's probably a word for that. Is it dogophile? Maybe it's beastophile. I did look it up once . . .'

'Do you spend much time online now, Layla?'

'No, I'm not allowed online. Which is a shame. Because I don't know how my virtual farm is doing. I should be checking every day and watering and stuff like that. But I did notice that, when I went on holiday, it did really well without me, so I hope it's okay . . .'

Her smooth forehead wrinkled like an older person's as she worried about her farm.

'Let's think about why you put the videos into categories,' I said. 'Is putting things in order important to you?'

Layla looked up again and nodded and something like her previous energy seemed to return.

'So how do you keep your socks at home? Do you just fling them into the drawer or –'

'No, of course not! All my clean socks are in order. They're arranged according to colour, or if they're sports socks . . . I mean, I hate netball but we have to do it. So, my socks are next to each other and then my tights and next to them are my pants. That's because I have three drawers.

Four would be good, but I only have three, so my socks and tights and pants have to share. It's socks on the left, tights in the middle, pants on the right. The next drawer down is T-shirts, and they're in colour order. And below that I put jeans, trousers, shorts . . . Mum makes me hang up my skirts.'

I asked: 'Do you wash your hands a lot?'

She considered this.

'Not really.'

'Or worry about your hands not being clean, or anything like that?'

'Not really.'

Layla had some obsessional symptoms, and the way she liked to order things was relevant. But she wasn't really hitting the threshold for obsessive compulsive disorder.

'Let's go back to the files. This Sadie person . . .'

As usual, Layla was helpful.

'Sadie3245.'

'Of course, Sadie might have been a made-up name – this person may have been a man, may have been twelve years old or fifty. Did Sadie ever reply to your messages and tell you anything about herself or himself?'

'No.'

'So what happened next?'

'I came home from school one day and the police were in the kitchen with my mother and she was crying. I just stood there and one of them walked up to me and said he was arresting me for possessing and distributing child pornography. I couldn't hear what he said next because Mum was howling so loudly. But I thought it must be to do with the files that Sadie3245 had sent me.'

'That must have been frightening.'

'I was really scared. I tried to tell them about ponies and how Sadie3245 had a palomino. But my mother was yelling: "Sadie, who the hell is this Sadie?" She was making such a noise, I couldn't explain. So the police took me in their car. I always used to think it would be sort of exciting in a police car with a blue flashing light but they didn't turn that on.'

'Did they take you to the police station?'

'Yes. They put me in a room and a lady from social services came in and then they asked me loads of questions, everyone did, oh, I think there was a nurse as well.'

It was through this case that I learned how the police monitored Dropbox activity, especially if they see strange, zipped files like the ones Layla received. Layla, with her love of order, passion for ponies and her online farm, was an innocent and easy target for Sadie3245, who I strongly suspected was a man with no ponies at all. The fact that any online paedophile might be expected to shield his Dropbox and re-route with VPN appeared to alter nothing for the police. To them, Layla's case looked open and shut.

33

Layla was a very unusual child. I felt she was vulnerable. But there was no clear-cut psychiatric case I could make for her. I nevertheless strongly believed that she should not be prosecuted. A combination of strong feelings and no evidence is a precursor to failure in court and, predictably, the prosecuting barrister ate me for breakfast.

As I got to know his face beneath his wig, I grew to hate his silky tone, his arrogance, his great certainty about a vulnerable child whose life the system was about to wreck. For him, Layla was just another case he would walk away from at the end of the day. It's hard to be sure about anything – in life, in psychiatry – but I was sure that this case should not be proceeding.

The prosecution barrister stood upright, looked at me and put his head on one side, as if he were carefully considering an object in a museum.

'Many people would not believe a young girl could be capable of committing such an offence but the evidence here is irrefutable. This girl has a twisted mind. She is, in fact, a menace to all innocent young children. Isn't she?'

'I do not believe you are right.'

'Your beliefs do not interest the court because the evidence is clear. The defendant not only watched this material, and many times, but she catalogued it under such headings as: *Girls, aged five to ten: crying. Girls, aged five to ten:*

not crying. You claim that she was driven by some deep-seated urge to categorize what she saw – although not, you say, at a level which is psychiatrically recognized. May I remind you that the *Girls, aged five to ten: crying* were at the time crying because they were being hideously sexually abused? Or are you claiming Layla didn't notice that?'

'I don't doubt that she knew what she was watching, but I am arguing that she had no sexual understanding or interest. Of course she was curious, in the same way that she might have been curious about a New Forest pony but –'

'Oh, really Dr Harding, please do not try to persuade the court that an academically gifted child like Layla does not know the difference between a New Forest pony and a girl who is being sexually abused.'

'I'm saying that Layla succumbed to morbid curiosity. How many of us have stared at a crash on the other side of the motorway, even though we really don't want to see dead bodies? Layla has few friends: she's quite socially isolated. And she clearly has difficulties understanding some of the social nuances of the world around her. I don't think she was sufficiently developed to have any sexual interest in the images. If she was, then she would have shielded her activity from scrutiny, the way real paedophiles do. Whoever sent her that link should be in the dock.'

I did not add that, along with Sadie3245, I'd like to put the prosecution barrister in the dock and the whole criminal justice system too. Here was a roomful of adults in fusty wigs passing easy judgement on a child because the system was unable to function with anything more complex that the binary notion of guilty or not guilty. And mental health is often a lot more complex than that.

'The incontrovertible evidence is that Layla watched extreme pornography and then renamed and organized the files. Correct?'

'Yes but –'

'And the prosecution's case is that renaming the files is a short step away from distributing them, for wider consumption.'

'But she didn't do that.'

'Her arrest came soon enough to prevent her preying on many innocent children, and that is not something we should regret, Dr Harding.'

'But I don't think –'

'Your thoughts and musings are simply not useful to the court. As a professional, you have had to admit that Layla has no mental impairment to mitigate her behaviour. You have stated this as fact, the only fact you have offered us, and the prosecution therefore has no further questions for the witness. Thank you.'

He sat down. The court was very quiet. Layla, from behind her Perspex screen, gave me a kind smile.

The defence barrister worked hard to redeem the situation.

'You have been asked, Dr Harding, to address the question of underlying health problems in order to help us understand what has happened here. What are your conclusions?'

I took a deep breath. I ached all over, as if I'd been set upon and beaten up. I turned to the jury.

'A lot of people around Layla have picked up that she's

a little bit different. As a result, she's been examined by professionals on a few occasions. The suspicion has been autistic spectrum disorder. But she's never quite reached the diagnostic threshold for that or any other defined condition. I concur with this. But I did find that she suffers from a diffuse neuropsychiatric syndrome. In other words, she presents with traits of a number of different conditions. In my view, she has particular vulnerabilities that make her very susceptible to negative influences online.'

'However, that is not in itself a mental health diagnosis?'

'Life doesn't always fit into neat diagnostic boxes. Many illnesses are on a continuum, they don't jump in and out of definitions to suit us. And although the defendant doesn't suffer from any particular mental illness, she does, in my view, suffer from a burden of diffuse illness traits. Online, anyone who already has difficulty understanding social cues and communication is at a particular disadvantage.'

'Dr Harding, how many children do you think, as a psychiatrist, that you have seen who are either the victims or the perpetrators or perhaps both, of child abuse?'

I was taken aback.

'Well . . . I don't know. I couldn't put a figure on that.'

'Ten, maybe? Twenty? Thirty?'

'Oh no, we're not talking about tens but hundreds.'

'You have seen hundreds of such children over the course of your career?'

'Certainly.'

'Then I feel sure that the court will recognize that your opinion is based on long training and wide experience. And it is your expert opinion that this child, Layla, did not know what she was doing when she downloaded this material. And that instead of taking a sexual interest in it, she simply responded as she might to any great muddle of material, and categorized it?'

'Yes, that is my opinion. She was deeply shocked by what she saw: that is what she told me and I believe her. In my view, she managed that distress by doing what she always does: sorting the material into categories. Making sense of it in her own particular way. This is a girl who categorizes everything, and particularly those things in the world that make her feel something. I haven't examined her computer myself, but she told me that she has folders on her desktop for each breed of native pony, divided into subcategories of colour, size and so on . . . lots of different parameters, in fact. I would suggest that Layla categorizing images that distress her is similar to Layla categorizing images, like ponies, that please her. She is overwhelmed by emotion and she places it within a more familiar, safer, psychological framework in order to understand it. I do not think that she intended to distribute the images. She was simply displaying a well-established trait of her unique character.'

It was the jury's job to decide which of two psychiatrists was right about Layla. The prosecution psychiatrist and I were presenting them with some very fine differences in diagnosis and some significant differences in interpretation.

Unfortunately, the prosecution case was much easier to understand than our complex, nuanced defence. Layla was found guilty and not allowed to return home.

I was angry for weeks. But I certainly did not expect to

see her again. She must have been released by now and be living with her mother again. So what could have happened? What could she have done a few years later that required the involvement of her solicitor and a psychiatrist once more? I badly wanted to know but first I had to go out of town. I had been asked to see a young person called Sally.

34

As the train sped west, the countryside seemed to thicken. When I alighted at a station, it was surrounded by trees and when the taxi took me to Sally's secure children's home I found it nestling in woodland in its own grounds. But there the fairy tale ended. Nearby was a housing estate where homes were painted in bright Farrow & Ball colours, but Sally's home was grey and dour. Its lawn was overgrown and its façade had not been painted for many years.

By now I had played a role in enough high-profile cases to very often be contacted by strangers for help. In Sally's case, there was evidently no criminal activity to address. Just a dilemma I was being asked to help resolve. The local services wanted advice from someone far away from their area who did not know Sally or any of the professionals involved.

Sally and her parents were waiting in the clean, plain family room. Sally was twelve but might easily be mistaken for a fourteen-year-old. She was tall and significantly overweight. She had dark eyes and long, dark hair with a thick fringe curving over her eyebrows. Her parents sat on either side. They seemed small and thin and worried. I banished quickly from my mind a most unwelcome and perhaps unkind image: of a cuckoo, sitting in the nest of two tiny and exhausted birds who were endeavouring to keep up with the demands of their immense baby.

Sally's mother remained seated when I entered. She held

Sally's hand and I saw her squeeze it comfortingly. Her father got up to greet me. Both parents were warm and friendly: in fact, they seemed pleased to see me. Sally made eye contact when I greeted her but said nothing. She pointed to a plate of biscuits on the table. Her mother offered me one politely and then gave one to Sally. Soon afterwards, Sally pointed again, and her mother gave her another.

She was unlucky enough to have been born to parents who had subjected her to extreme neglect and abuse. She had been removed from them at the age of three and had remained in foster care until, when she was nine, this brave couple had adopted her. Brave because, in the previous six years, Sally had been fostered no fewer than six times. Every placement had broken down, always for the same reason. Sally was violent.

Her nice and well-meaning adoptive parents were the sort of exceptional, principled people who had decided not to bring any more children into a crowded world but to devote themselves instead to a disadvantaged child. They truly believed that all the cuddles and love they had to offer could make up for Sally's early traumas and help her lead a fulfilling life. I was glad that such good people existed and I admired them for their efforts.

The father was an accountant and company director. The mother had been a speech therapist but had given up her job to take care of Sally. I knew their ages, and they both looked considerably older. Their three years with Sally had, I suspected, exhausted them.

When we were seated, I looked at Sally and started by introducing a subject I knew would make her feel comfortable: her love of animals and the farm she sometimes visited.

'There are lambs,' she told me. 'I like the lambs best.'

No mention of ponies yet, then.

'Do you give them names?'

'I like one called Chocolate.'

'Did you give him that name?'

'Yes, Chocolate is just the same colour as a bar of Cadbury's Dairy Milk.'

I smiled. So far so good. We continued to talk about animals and she engaged with this and answered appropriately; in fact, she was so docile that it was hard to believe all that I had learned about her. Because her notes said that, when Sally was violent, she didn't just throw her toys across the room. No, she set out to harm people with scissors, knives, stones, bricks, broken glass, china, anything that might hurt them. However, her parents understood her traumatic past and this enabled them to respond to her attacks not with anger but with forgiveness. Not with stern rules but with loving acceptance.

Being middle-class, articulate and expecting help to be available, they soon found their way to the Child and Adolescent Mental Health Service and were asking for assessments and support.

They were convinced that Sally must be autistic. In fact, she did not meet the threshold for autism but it seemed that word was never far away when people discussed her. And a lot of professionals were now discussing her. The heart of the problem, everyone said, was Sally's early years' trauma.

Suddenly Sally sat up straight and made an announcement: 'I'm going to give a performance.'

'Oh, are you going to dance for Dr Harding?' asked her father. His tone exuded enthusiasm and gratitude, as if a prima ballerina had just dropped by and agreed to go *en pointe* for some adoring fans.

'Wonderful!' exclaimed her mother.

'I expect everyone would like to watch the performance,' Sally said, getting back on her feet in a lumbering fashion that did not remind me of a dancer at all.

Her father picked up the cue.

'I'm sure they would!' he enthused, rushing off to fetch the carers.

Three smiling women came in, two of them pushed the sofa out of the way, and I was asked to shuffle my chair back a few feet.

'Is the music ready?' asked Sally. Her father was already stationed by an old-fashioned record player in the corner.

'We think vinyl gives the best quality sound,' her mother explained quietly: our chairs were close now, to give Sally maximum performance space. 'Sally loves it.'

Sally said: 'Quiet please, while I concentrate.'

Total silence fell on the room. She struck a pose. One leg pointed out and she attempted, rather unsuccessfully, to balance on the other. An arm was raised – not sinuously, but more like someone trying to hail a bus.

We all waited. I wished the music would start, because what had begun as a small wobble was now escalating into violent shaking. The pose was in imminent danger of collapse.

'Almost ready!' cried her father from the corner.

Suddenly, loudly, the room was filled with the grandeur of Beethoven's Fifth.

Da da da DUM.

Sally leapt into action. From her pose she exploded into something like a star jump. She paused when the music did and then created a second pose. And as the music became more fluent, so did she, galloping heavily from side to side, shaking the floorboards, thumping like thunder, throwing arms haphazardly in all directions, her facial expression showing how seriously she took this display.

As she puffed, grunted and banged her way through one of the world's greatest pieces of music, I glanced around at the others. They looked enraptured.

'Bravo!' cried her mother as Sally's feet created an exceptionally loud crash by landing squarely on the ground together, causing the record player, not for the first time, to screech and jump a few bars. Sally's performance was not affected by this hiccough in her musical accompaniment. She lurched through a particularly alarming twirl and the carers burst into what seemed like spontaneous applause.

'Does Sally have ballet lessons?' I murmured to her mother.

She smiled and shook her head fondly, without taking her eyes off her daughter. 'Sally wouldn't have the patience for lessons.'

Sally's impatience with lessons of all kinds had been mentioned in her notes. She had been expelled from a whole list of primary schools for violent behaviour and had eventually been given a home tutor. Whom Sally had attacked. Lessons had ended then, but now they had resumed.

At last her father stopped the music. The dancer, red-faced and sweating, finished with a final flourish.

There was a moment's silence. Then the whole room erupted into applause. Sally curtsied as her audience clapped, whooped and yelled. One of the carers called for an encore, but everyone could see that Sally was too exhausted to repeat the performance.

It seemed churlish not to clap, but how could I collude with a roomful of people who were assuring Sally that we had just seen something sensational? Her dancing was a cartoon, a caricature, and they must surely realize that. And yet everyone was keen to indulge her.

For a few minutes we rearranged the chairs again, Sally flopping into one while her carers rushed for a cold drink.

Mother hugged daughter. 'I'm so proud of you,' she said.

Sally had come close to killing both her adoptive parents on various occasions and, for their safety, six months ago she had been removed from their home. When it was generally agreed that, although not actually autistic, she had neuro-developmental difficulties, a council care package was opened for her.

She was placed in community care and given extensive social services support. Unfortunately, that placement had ended when she attacked a carer. Another placement ended similarly. And in the next home, something terrible happened.

There had been an argument with a carer one Friday evening. But on Saturday Sally seemed to have forgotten it and was, by all accounts, calm and friendly. She laughed and joked with all the staff. And then went into the kitchen, where she boiled a kettle of water. She called for help when the carer she had argued with was just outside the room. As soon as the carer entered, Sally was ready with a pan of the boiled water. She threw it directly into the woman's face, burning and partly blinding her victim. The carer had not worked since.

I had read about this incident in detail. It seemed to me that it had been premeditated and planned. That is, instrumental in nature, rather than reactive. The distinction between instrumental violence and reactive violence is absolutely critical to establish in such cases. The tendency of the world around a vulnerable child is to think that all violence must be reactive – even if reacting to long-ago developmental trauma. But I am not always in agreement with this assumption and it seemed to me that Sally's violence on that occasion had been planned. Thought out. Instrumental.

The police were called. No charges were pressed. Instead Sally was now detained under the Children Act and transferred, against her will, to this children's secure unit. Where it was found, once again, that she did not present with any mental disorder.

Sally's case was at the heart of some searching questions. How does a civilized society deal with children who express such violence? How can we afford the huge expense associated with this? Is it possible that a child can behave this way and *not* be mentally ill? And if not ill enough for treatment, how might detention in a psychiatric unit for the mentally ill, where she would live with the distressed and the psychotic, influence the intensity and complexity of her own behaviour?

It was clear to all that, whoever looked after her, a high level of care would be required: Sally could not safely be let loose in the world. The local mental health team, who had already assessed her, recommended that she continue under the care of social services, and that a bespoke community placement would be needed when she left the secure children's home. This bespoke placement might be a house, but it would need to be locked and heavily staffed until the risk that Sally posed to others lessened.

I daresay that the local authority was reluctant to take on this enormous expense and was hoping to hear that actually Sally was mentally ill and could live in a secure mental health unit. And that was where I came in. I had been asked to give an objective opinion on the huge question: who should take care of Sally?

I noted how the pendulum had swung from social care to health care, propelled partly by Sally's violence, and also by the assumption of family and professionals that she must have an illness that could be treated. Here was a vulnerable child. A child who was already being cared for by the state and who had suffered unspeakable traumas in her short life. But with no diagnosed mental disorder, the pendulum was now swinging back to social care.

The secure unit seemed to be both calm and well-run. There was apparently only one other child in this wing and she kept herself hidden away in her room for much of the time. So Sally received a lot of attention and support from the home's trained professionals. They catered for her every need as best they could. They aimed to keep her safe and to help her heal from her traumatic past, no matter how difficult she was.

Right now, Sally appeared relaxed after her dancing. We resumed the interview – until there was a loud noise outside the room. Evidently the authorities had noticed that overgrown lawn. And they had decided to cut it right now.

Sally leapt to her feet. I noticed her mother flinch – a small but instinctive gesture. I wondered how often Sally had jumped up to hit her.

She looked wildly about and, even when she had received many assurances that this was simply a lawn mower, she would not sit down without going to another room to check. Her mother went with her.

As soon as they were out of earshot, her father turned to me. He spoke softly and urgently.

'We don't know exactly what happened to Sal when she was a baby. Certainly she was neglected and went hungry: I'm afraid that . . .' His voice dropped further. '. . . she was probably sexually abused. And now we have a terrible problem. We hope you can help us. Sal started with Facebook about six months ago and almost immediately her biological mother found her there. She won't stop contacting her!'

I looked at him with concern.

'Can you do anything? That woman has caused no end of disruption and I'm sure that a lot of Sal's recent violence is entirely due to –'

He broke off as Sally returned, her mother close behind her. They sat down. Sally held a couple more biscuits in her hand. The mother smiled at me to continue the interview.

'I love to dance and to sing,' Sally told me while she munched. 'I'll give you another performance later.'

'When do you most like to dance?' I asked her. 'Perhaps when you're feeling happy? Or sad?'

She shrugged and did not reply.

'I know you do get very upset and overwhelmed,' I said. 'Do you ever dance when you feel that way?'

'No. I don't.'

I changed approach.

'When you're at the farm, do you ever hurt the animals you told me about? Have you ever hurt Chocolate?'

She shook her head so vigorously that her hair flew around her face in a manner reminiscent of her performance.

'I would never hurt any animal. I love them.'

'How would you feel,' I asked, 'if someone else hurt an animal?'

'Very sad. Because we should look after animals,' she informed me gravely.

'How do you cope if you feel overwhelmed when you are near an animal on the farm?'

'If I'm having a shouty I just walk away.'

'What are you thinking about at times like that?'

'I am thinking I must not frighten the rabbits because a rabbit can die of fright.'

'Do you think the same thing when you are upset or overwhelmed around people?'

'No.'

'What happens, Sally, when you have a shouty?' I asked curiously. 'Do you shout a lot?'

'Not always. Sometimes I hurt myself. Sometimes I hurt other people.'

Her father leaned towards me. 'There's a cycle of events. Sal has a shouty and gets violent. The police come. They Section her and take her to the Child and Adolescent

Mental Health Service. Later that day, the police bring her back. This can happen over and over and over again.'

He spoke evenly but I thought that in his voice I heard quiet desperation. I could almost visualize the pendulum swinging to the police, over to mental health services, then back to the family. Rinse and repeat. I glanced at his wife. She was still seated but her eyes were closed now. Sally was occupied and for just a few moments she could relax.

I turned back to Sally. 'So the police come and Section you and then they bring you back when you're calm. Is there any way this cycle could be broken?'

Her shrug was helpless. 'No. It just has to play itself out.'

'Sal doesn't have shouties with us like she used to,' her mother said, 'but she does with the carers. They can't take her outside unless it's three to one. In case she starts.'

'Sally needs three carers to go outside?'

Her parents nodded and glanced at Sally, who had heard all this. Now she sighed expressively: 'Yeeees.' As if we were talking about someone else, someone over whom she had no control.

We discussed the secure unit.

'What's the worst thing that's happened since you've been here?' I asked.

'Well, I had a big shouty once and I suppose there were problems when I jumped in front of that car.'

'Were you thinking that you wanted to hurt yourself when you did that?'

'I wasn't really thinking straight. Part of me wanted to hurt myself and part of me didn't.'

Her father said: 'Sal's been in hospital a few times. She swallowed a bottle of drain cleaner once . . .'

'And she did eat quite a lot of nail varnish,' added the mother.

Sally shuffled restlessly in her seat. Was a shouty imminent? Her mother immediately gave her a biscuit.

'See, Sal's shouties come out of the blue and if you're not ready for them or trained to deal with them they can be a bit of a shock,' said the father. 'You can think you're getting on really well and then suddenly . . .' He made a big gesture with his hands, like an explosion.

'What do you experience, Sally, when you have a shouty?' I asked.

She shrugged. 'Sometimes I don't know what's going on. I don't know how to control it.'

Her mother looked sad. 'The police do quite often have to restrain her.'

'And, there's medication,' added her father.

I asked Sally: 'Do you only hurt people when you feel overwhelmed and have a shouty? Or do you sometimes plan to hurt them?'

'Maybe once a month I plan to hurt someone.'

'Can you tell me more?'

She could not. I thought of her planned attack with the boiling water. The notes said that she had feigned friendship so that the carer would feel safe entering the room alone with her – and then Sally had launched her assault. Maybe her mother was thinking of that too. She looked sad and defeated. She said: 'Sometimes Sally hides something sharp, maybe a piece of broken glass, and then she comes back to use it later: on herself or, more often, others.'

'Have you ever been charged with assault, Sally?' I asked.

'I've been arrested.'

Her father said: 'Sal has never been charged.'

'I read how you cut your mother with a blade. Were you charged then?'

All three of them shook their heads vehemently.

'We don't want to criminalize a traumatized child and neither do the police,' said her mother. 'They often arrest her and she calms down when she's handcuffed. When they've got her to the CAMHS hub, they de-arrest her.'

'None of these violent incidents has ever been processed by the police?'

The mother looked shocked at the suggestion. 'Oh no, I don't think anyone believes that's the right way to go about things with someone so vulnerable.'

'We have always approached Sal's problems with love and understanding,' her father told me. 'We feel love will win through.'

Assessing her empathy, I said: 'Sally, I'm wondering how you feel after a shouty, when you've hurt your mother or father?'

She paused.

'Well, a little bit sad,' she admitted.

'When you see that people are upset, does that make you feel very sorry? Maybe you say you're sorry?'

'No,' she said. 'I don't think so.' She stretched and yawned. 'I'm going to sing now.'

Her parents expressed delight but my heart sank. I hoped it wouldn't be as awkward as her dancing.

We dutifully rearranged our chairs while her father went to the record player. The carers came in and stood in a row. Sally waited, her head bowed in concentration before her performance. I glanced at the clock.

'Sally's going to sing: "Walking in the Air" from *The Snowman*,' her father announced in a big voice as if he was introducing her at the Palladium. The backing music started and I braced myself.

But now Sally surprised me. Her voice was lovely! It was pure and silvery as it soared to the highest notes, fell, then rose again. She sounded like an angel. That song has the power to move and Sally's young voice, lingering on some notes, dancing over others, was certainly moving. I listened, enraptured, understanding now how everyone was so ready to love her and feel compassion for her. It seemed her singing came from some deep, sweet place within her. It must be easy for those around her to believe they were accessing the true Sally when she sang.

'*. . . swimming in the fro-zen sky . . .*'

And then, a phone rang.

The singing stopped. The music continued. And the electronic chirruping of the phone was clearly audible over it. Sally's eyes widened. Her body seemed to expand, as if she was filling with air.

'Whoops, sorry, I thought I'd switched it off!' cried a carer, exiting rapidly to the hallway.

Sally emitted a long, high-pitched scream, her mouth huge, her eyes blazing, her face red with fury. She rushed, still screaming, behind the carer, leaving the music without a singer and the room without its star. I could hear her loudly yelling obscenities and feared for the carer's safety, but the other carers were not far behind, and, from the sound of it, they were trying to restrain Sally. The music stopped and now I could distinguish some of the cries between her high-pitched screams: 'My fucking performance! You bitch, you bitch, your fucking phone ruined it, you fucking bitch . . .'

Her parents looked uncomfortable.

'We've been told not to intervene,' her father said, looking as if he really did not want to intervene anyway. After their years of violence from Sally, it must feel good to leave her so-called shouties to the professionals.

'Sorry about this, Doctor,' said her mother. 'She's been so much worse since this social media thing started with her biological family. It was right after the mother first made contact that she blinded the carer. We'd welcome any help you can give. The mother won't go away. You've no idea what a worry it is. She's a deliberately mischievous woman, always putting ideas into Sally's head.'

She stopped talking and put her head in her hands.

The father showed me screengrabs on his phone of the kind of messages the biological mother was leaving. Inviting Sally to see her, reply, live with her. Saying that she had never wanted to lose her, that Sally had been taken against her will, that her adoptive parents did not love her and only kept her for the money they were paid.

I said: 'Oh, this is really unhelpful.'

'We know she had other children taken away – is she doing this with all of them?' asked the father. 'She has to be stopped.'

The messages certainly seemed designed to disrupt Sally's relationship with her parents. I could understand how easily this might affect Sally's behaviour, as well as leading the kind couple to despair.

Her father said: 'We know you're here to write a report about where Sally should live, but if you could mention the problem with this woman . . . we're trying to get social services to have her blocked by court order and anything you can say will help.'

I nodded.

'I'm so sorry that you're having to cope with this. I'll have to consider it carefully, and will read all the information, but I don't think Sally having contact with her biological family is helpful. And certainly not now. But we can't deflect all of Sally's problems on to this woman's arrival on Facebook. Sally was violent before her biological mother appeared on the scene, wasn't she? And there's nothing new about her shouties?'

The angry yells from outside the room had subsided now. A carer entered, red faced, dishevelled, smoothing her hair after the rigours of restraining Sally.

She looked at me and said apologetically: 'I'm afraid Sally won't come back in.'

'Have you tried giving her a biscuit?' asked her mother, weakly.

'She threw it in my face. And she says she won't continue the interview. Would you like to wait to see if she changes her mind?'

'No thanks,' I said. 'I think I've seen enough to write my report.'

35

The train rushed east in the dimming evening light. It was August and the grass was long and trees were heavy with leaves, with pollen, with summer. How beautiful the world seemed and how sad that Sally could never experience the outdoors alone or with a loved one but only accompanied by three vigilant carers. Hers was perhaps a joyless existence.

Generally I carry out collateral interviews after, not before, seeing a child, in case the interviews prejudice me. But this time there had been no choice as so many people were heading off on holiday.

When I had phoned Sally's social worker, she had been very keen to speak. She told me that Sally was her most complex case – and in many ways her most worrying. Sally's violence was getting worse and worse, the staff turnover among her carers was very high, and it was hard to place her. Sometimes her violence was sudden, when she seemed to lose control, but not always.

'We feel sure that there really must be mental health issues here,' she told me, 'and that she should be in mental health care.'

'Does Sally ever plan violence?' I asked.

'Oh yes, definitely; she can be very calculating in her cruelty, planning all sorts of ways to hurt people. She's quite a problem.'

Mrs Polly, who was manager of the unit, said that the staff often suspected Sally was violent in order to gain attention from the police or the hospital. They were currently trying not to call 999 to avoid reinforcing her behaviour.

'Can you give me an example,' I asked, 'of an occasion when Sally has deliberately planned to be violent since she arrived in your unit?'

'Oh, I can think of a lot! Let's see, what about the things she did to poor Gloria? Gloria, of all people, one of our best carers. She slipped out with the rubbish in the pouring rain and Sally was at the door when she tried to get back in and managed to really slam it on her hand.'

'That sounds terrible. Did she do much harm?'

'Gloria was badly bruised and almost lost her finger. She needed surgery.'

'Did she press charges?'

'Oh no. She just asked to be moved. All our carers are trained and understand that this challenging behaviour is coming from a bad place and it isn't really Sally's fault.'

I asked: 'Do you think Sally feels remorse after she's hurt someone? Especially if she's fond of them?' I was remembering the reports which said that, while still living at home, she had attacked her mother with a hammer and tried to push her father out of an upstairs window.

'No. I don't think she ever feels bad.'

'Does she express regret?'

'No. Her parents made her write a letter to Gloria which was a sort of apology. But in general she won't ever say sorry.'

'Do you believe she considers how it must feel for

people to be attacked by her? For her dad to know that she tried to push him out of a window?'

'No, I don't. She has no empathy, that's for sure. I wouldn't really expect it, after a tough start like that in life.'

Finally, I spoke to Sally's consultant psychiatrist.

'She's quite a challenge. Every provider in the area is running out of carers who'll work with her,' said Dr Weaver.

'Does anyone ever think of pressing charges when she hurts them?'

'Of course not! Who would want to criminalize her?'

'What's your diagnosis?'

'Well, there's the difficulty. She doesn't strictly meet diagnostic criteria for any mental illness. The closest might be some kind of post-traumatic stress disorder, though she doesn't present with the classical features. I know a lot of people suggest that she has autistic spectrum disorder, but I don't think Sally's clinically autistic. Although if you told me there are some neuro-developmental vulnerabilities, I'd agree with you. But basically her emotional dysregulation – what she calls her "shouties" – can be explained entirely by developmental trauma. I presume you know about her early years?'

Yes, everyone had been keen to tell me. They seemed to define Sally by the first few years of her life.

As the train cut through the countryside and darkness fell across the world gently like a net, I thought about my own diagnosis of Sally.

Her hypervigilance when the mower had started outside was the one behaviour I had witnessed that did seem to confirm Dr Weaver's suspicion of PTSD, although, like her, I could find no other evidence of this disorder. I did not think Sally was autistic, although I agreed that she showed some neuro-developmental traits.

I did feel, however, that there could be some concerning emerging aspects of her personality. Twelve is far too young to consider a personality disorder diagnosis, but emerging traits of personality are worth noting, as these can develop into further difficulties in adulthood. Although Sally was clearly a vulnerable child, aspects of her challenging behaviours and personality structure met the diagnostic criteria for an unsocialized conduct disorder. Rather than being an underlying illness that results in bad behaviours, this diagnosis describes a constellation of antisocial and challenging behaviours. Alongside her lack of empathy and apparently callous disregard for the feelings and safety of others, a conduct disorder implied that if she continued on this trajectory she might develop into an antisocial adult. And in some cases, particularly those demonstrating callous and unemotional traits, such disorders can ultimately develop into psychopathy.

Once the world outside the train was entirely obliterated by the night, I fished my laptop out of my bag and began to type my report.

I agreed with Dr Weaver that Sally didn't present with signs or symptoms of mental disorder, and that she did not suffer from chronic or enduring mental illness. And with no mental disorder, Sally could not be detained under the Mental Health Act. So, the possibility of being cared for long-term in a secure mental health unit was off the table, and I felt this wouldn't be good for her anyway. Without an illness to treat, how could she ever be safely released? She could find herself stuck there. Her needs were complex and she required a high degree of support and care – but in the community, not in a locked psychiatric unit.

I supported the parents' efforts to stop Sally's biological mother from contacting her because it could only lead to further confusion for Sally. This was particularly the case now, when she was twelve years old and so much was changing for her. I described my concerns around her emerging personality structure, suggesting long-term talking therapies that might help her stave off her violent and debilitating personality traits.

I confined to just a few lines something that I felt strongly about:

> *In my opinion, some of Sally's violence is planned and intentional. In my view she has a degree of autonomy regarding her actions and should therefore face the normal social consequences for purposive violence. These consequences may include the involvement of youth justice in her care and management in the community, alongside health and social care. In my view, understanding that she must face consequences for her actions may help her accept a degree of responsibility for them, and could help her adapt her behaviour and thereby improve her long-term wellbeing.*

It was well-hidden in a detailed report, but I knew that brief paragraph would jump out at Sally's parents like a headline. They would read it with horror. And her social worker, Mrs Polly, Dr Weaver and perhaps all her carers would be just as shocked. Mrs Polly had said that no one pressed charges because they believed that Sally's behaviour was not her fault. But I was ready to defend my view and knew I would probably have to.

As soon as I was home, I sounded off to Hazel. She was chopping vegetables in the kitchen.

Ignoring our agreement not to talk about our work, I said: 'You wouldn't believe it. This girl suddenly announced she was going to give a performance and then she thumped around pretending to be a ballet dancer.'

'That's not such a strange thing for a child to do,' Hazel said. She was busy and did not look at me.

'But we were all supposed to join in this idea that she's a brilliant ballerina and clap and whoop at the end!'

Hazel seemed unfazed.

'She's a child, it's nice to encourage her.'

'I'm all for encouraging children to find their voice and passion in life, but this was collusion. They tiptoe around her all the time. Whenever she thought the girl might kick off, the mother gave her a biscuit.'

I paused for the hiss and sizzle of the pan. And then continued.

'It seemed there weren't any boundaries. They simply tolerated her challenging behaviour from the beginning because they were being understanding. When they first adopted her, she was a traumatized child who was acting out so they were kind. They continued to accommodate her as she got older, even when she became violent. Now she gets to twelve and she's very violent indeed and the situation is made far worse when the biological mother contacts her on Facebook. But hey, now they can blame the biological mother for all the recent behaviour. It's still not the girl's fault and they continue to show love and tolerance and understanding by agreeing to her every wish and throwing her biscuits.'

'What are the parents like?'

'Wonderful and kind and they have deep concerns about this girl's early traumas. The trauma history isn't clear, but they hold on to it. They seem terrified by it. When she went out of the room, her father leaned forward and whispered to me that it was thought someone had sexually abused her. How much of that terror is projected on to the child, even unconsciously? How does she make sense of that? Don't get me wrong, these parents were the best and I don't blame them for anything. But I've seen it before. Some adoptive parents can hold their children's trauma and keep it alive for them. Then it can be unconsciously and very subtly projected on to the child. As though something is terribly wrong in the world, but the child can't work out exactly what it is.'

We were sitting down to eat now. Spicy aromas wafted from my plate.

'This looks delicious,' I said. 'But the point is, children are sponges. They absorb so much from their parents, so much that is conscious and unconscious. And in Sally's case, the parents know all about the elephant in the room: past sexual abuse.'

Hazel said: 'Duncan, you won't criticize her parents in your report, will you?'

'Nope. But they'll hate it anyway. Instead of the police just arriving and restraining her and being gentle and taking their helmets off so they don't frighten her, she needs a police liaison officer who will help to contain her – not drop her like a hot potato once she's de-arrested and in healthcare. She's stabbing people! Why have the health system and social care been left to pick up the pieces? With such risk, why hasn't the criminal justice system been involved in her management?'

'She's only twelve.'

'True, but the next few years will fly by. And at this rate, something very serious will occur. Actually, there's already been some serious violence; she just hasn't been charged for it. The assumption is that this is all trauma, and that it can somehow be hugged away. Or treated away. They are all assuming that she isn't responsible for her violence. But I'm afraid in my view she is. And if she's stabbing people, she needs professionals working with her who are expert in that. Health and social care are totally out of their depth with it. Youth justice, the criminal justice system: knife crime is something they deal with all the time.'

'You're God's gift to all those lock 'em up types. They'll adopt you for a mascot.'

'But I'm not one of them! I really think this is for the child's own good. She's a complex girl who needs a complex support network. If she's charged and convicted, she'll be managed in part by the Youth Offending Service. They're brilliant at dealing with her sort of violence – in a criminal, not a health context. They can manage that risk. It could be the best thing to happen to her.'

Hazel shook her head. 'I somehow don't think her loving parents will buy into that. They won't want her criminalized.'

'I hear that a lot,' I said. 'But with this level of violence, she's really criminalizing herself. The violence will progress. It's already progressing. And eventually something really terrible will happen. She needs a clear boundary now. And that boundary needs to be built up and reinforced with the help of the police and youth justice. They can't just wash their hands of her. She needs to be held.'

'So you're saying . . .' Hazel's tone told me that she had often heard me banging on about this. 'You're saying she's violent because she's been given no boundaries.'

'Well, that's one reason she's violent and that's one thing that can be changed. This is what goes wrong for so many of the kids I see. In my view, childhood is complicated enough to negotiate. We need to help by giving kids a solid framework. A societal framework, with normal consequences. If you choose to stab someone, you need to face the consequences of that behaviour. It can't be hugged away or treated away with medication. We must face the unpleasant truth that children can choose to do bad things. These behaviours should be acknowledged and contained by society. Boundaries are something we all need. A baby will keep kicking until it feels the edge of the cot.'

She half smiled. But only half. 'For a man with no baby, you seem to know a lot about them.'

Since I had returned home, the air had been filled with the sound of my voice. And now there was complete silence.

I looked at her. And then down at my plate. It was empty.

'Did you enjoy your meal?'

Oh no. And I hadn't even asked Hazel how she was. I had arrived with Sally inside my head and she had stayed there, filling the room with her atrocious dancing and her shouties. Now, what was that golden rule Ari Good had told me about so long ago? Was I really still ignoring it?

36

I woke early and finished my report on Sally. Then lobbed it west. I thought there would probably be shrapnel but not for a few weeks. It was time now to interview Callum once again. Remembering our last meeting, I half wished I hadn't promised.

First, I read the notes and watched the unsavoury CCTV footage Will had sent of Callum beating up one boy and then shooting the other.

He and his mates had surrounded the boys in an alleyway by a shop and Callum was calm throughout as he punched the first boy repeatedly and then smashed him against the wall. His victim dropped down the brickwork like a small, fluttering bird. This was the opposite of family viewing. The boy's utter terror. Callum's effortless punches. The way the other lad rushed forward and Callum simply reached for his gun as calmly as if he was reaching for a bottle of Evian water. It seemed to me that he smiled as he fired it.

Callum was not frenzied. He was not out of control.

It was chilling footage.

Will had tried to present Callum's action as gang warfare, and there was certainly an element of that, but it was hard to see Callum's mates as a tough gang. Their reluctance to participate in the fight was palpable. At least one of them looked as scared as the victims.

I learned that, remarkably, the victims were healing. The boy with the broken bones was walking. The kid with the gunshot wound was back at school and showing his mates the scar. But that had no bearing on the case for me. Callum had been a hair's breadth from killing one, perhaps two people and, if he had now found a way to acquire firearms, it seemed that no one was safe.

And so to Callum's interview. This time we met at a secure unit. There was little furniture but Callum still contrived not to look at me. He kept his hood up. When he finally spoke, he said: 'I told you before that you're a spaz dickhead, so why are you here being a spaz dickhead again?'

Things did not get much better after that.

I was soon worrying about the validity of the ADHD diagnosis, about how this young person was being labelled as vulnerable and ill. Especially as I myself had now watched him batter and shoot two people. It was one thing diagnosing ADHD in a primary school child like Benjamin and quite another in an aggressive adolescent with a long criminal record. And by now I was sure that this medical label had given everyone, including me, false hope for change in Callum's behaviour.

This time, I wrote in my report:

Callum has been arrested and charged on multiple occasions in the past. The view of professionals working with him was that he was suffering from a mental disorder, namely ADHD, that mitigated his responsibility for his criminal activities and violence.

Having considered this case carefully, I do not share this view. In my opinion, Callum does not present with overt signs and symptoms of mental disorder, and while he has been previously diagnosed with ADHD and childhood trauma, in my view these are not the primary drivers of his antisocial behaviours and violence towards others. In my view, his violent behaviours are an expression of his antisocial attitudes to life and those around him. I believe he retains a substantial degree of autonomy and responsibility for his actions.

It is possible that ADHD was misdiagnosed because its symptoms can easily be confused with the chaotic, impulsive behaviour of young people involved in crime and violence. It would be helpful if this diagnosis could be confirmed by professionals, though I understand that he has so far refused to engage with professionals in the community setting. It may be that a custodial setting is required in order for his mental health status to be properly assessed. In my opinion, Callum meets diagnostic criteria for conduct disorder, and he also presents with callous and unemotional personality traits.

For the second time in twenty-four hours, I diagnosed that possible precursor to psychopathy, conduct disorder.

I concluded:

I am extremely concerned about the risk Callum poses to other people. In my view, from my examination of the evidence available to me, this risk is significantly escalating. Previous community orders do not appear to have been effective in derailing his current trajectory of increasing risk. Nor do they seem to have significantly improved the quality of his life. He has not engaged with mental health services, although several professionals have tried to offer treatment and support.

At this point, I am of the view that without physical containment, i.e., detention in custody or in a secure social or healthcare setting, Callum's violence towards others will continue and could result in serious injury or death. I do not state this lightly. Physical containment would also be helpful in allowing health professionals to thoroughly assess Callum, and to provide any potential support or treatment that he may need.

About ten minutes after I finished the report and pressed send, the phone rang.

Will said: 'Duncan, this isn't what I was hoping for.'

'Sorry, Will. I know you'll want to put my report in the bin and find someone who says nicer things. But I have to be honest and I think it helps Callum too.'

'I can't put it in the bin. Not if you really think he could kill someone,' Will said miserably.

'That's a strong possibility. It's better to take action now than wait for a victim to die, or it would be on both our consciences. I already feel bad enough about the kid he shot in the alleyway. If I hadn't allowed a misplaced trust in ADHD medication to divert me then –'

Will interrupted. 'Duncan. Is Callum a psychopath?'

I hesitated. 'I don't describe anyone under eighteen as a psychopath. That would be stigmatizing them for life when there is still a chance of change before they become adults. But I mentioned conduct disorder. And that means there are indications psychopathy might emerge later.'

Will said: 'Doubt there's going to be a turn-around any time soon, but you never know.'

By advocating that Callum stayed locked up, I was certainly giving him the best chance of change. But by now I had accepted that, even in children, change was sometimes impossible. I remembered how Thomas the serial killer had been described by the prosecution as evil. I still did not believe in evil. Because if change was sometimes impossible, I had also seen that it was sometimes possible, in even the most hopeless cases. No, I would not use the word 'evil'. Not even about Callum.

It was a short tube ride to the cafe where I had been directed to meet Parminder Sharp, not far from her office. It was across the street from one of the big London hospitals and near a mainline station and there was a continual flow of people, past its windows, through its doors.

Parminder was there before me. She had succeeded in finding a table and was cradling a coffee in manicured hands. We greeted each other warmly. I remembered that Layla had compared her to a Dartmoor pony and this, coming from Layla, was a compliment.

'I'd better tell you what's been going on before we go into the hospital.' Her face creased a little. 'You're not going to like it.'

I fetched a tea and sat down. I could not imagine what Layla had done to upset this experienced solicitor so much.

'She hasn't done anything,' Parminder assured me, and I felt relief. But only for a moment.

'This time, Layla is a victim.'

'In my view, she's always been a victim.'

'She's been attacked. I need you to assess whether she should appear in court to give evidence in person against her attacker. I'm arguing for video only.'

'What's happened, for heaven's sake?'

'She was picked on and beaten up by a group of older girls. They were calling her a paedophile. They videoed the whole thing and posted it on social media. It looks really terrible. Unfortunately, no one was actually taking a picture when one of them ran forward and stabbed her.'

I felt as if this news had run forward and stabbed me, too. I gasped: 'No!'

'Oh yes. She's on the mend. I mean, she's off the ward and in paediatric recuperation. But.' Outside, the eddies of staff and patients and visitors and passengers swirled continuously. We watched them without seeing them. 'But.'

I still could not speak, the news was so shocking.

Parminder said: 'These were very nasty girls and they decided to do some very nasty things to her. On the grounds that she's a paedophile.'

'But . . . Layla's really not a paedophile!'

'Duncan, we lost the case. A jury found her guilty.'

'They never should have done!'

'Agreed.'

Parminder was trying to be cool and detached. I did not even attempt that. 'The case was a disgrace. It just gave the police a positive internet crime statistic. But all they did was use their expert digital skills to monitor unshielded Dropbox traffic and catch a kid. They completely missed the actual paedophile who sent that material in the first place. And –'

Now Parminder, too, had stopped sounding calm.

'Monstrous!' she cried. 'Monstrous. Of all my cases, this one still makes my blood boil.'

People were glancing up from their drinks and laptops at us, but we were so angry we didn't care.

'Because it was little more than a witch-hunt. And now, a bunch of horrible, scary girls have decided to look like rough justice superheroes!'

'They're not superheroes, they're just bullies,' Parminder said.

'Oh, the harm bullies can do. That poor kid.'

We were silent for a moment.

'If only,' Parminder said, 'Layla didn't keep identifying herself so openly as a paedophile.'

'That's because she's neurodiverse and the court told her she was a paedophile and all that treatment she had afterwards was for paedophiles and –'

'I just wish she hadn't been so honest about it. I mean, going around calling herself a sex offender. In her community, word gets out pretty quickly. I doubt this was the first time she was bullied.'

I felt sickened. 'What did they do to her?'

She sighed. 'Waited for her outside school and dragged her into some sort of alley, although frankly they were easy enough to see from the road and someone should have stopped them. But no one did. So they pulled most of her clothes off and hit her, hard, scratched her and burned her with matches, frightened and intimidated her, videoed it all . . . and then suddenly one of them produced a knife and stabbed her.'

I groaned.

'Just once?'

'In the lower abdomen. Very low indeed. You don't want to know what the bully was shouting when she did it.'

No. I didn't want to know what she was shouting.

'How bad's the damage? Physically, I mean.'

'Her reproductive organs have been severely hurt.'

'So she might not be able to have children?'

'I understand it's unlikely.'

I tried to imagine this happening to the sweet young girl I had known. I could not.

'The police have finally agreed to consult you about whether she's fit to testify in person at the attacker's trial. It took them a while to work out which girl it was, but she's admitted to the crime now. Then it took forever for the police to agree that you could assess Layla. And the trial's actually next week.'

'The girl is more likely to be found guilty if Layla appears.'

'She shouldn't appear.' Parminder stood up. 'We have to go now, I've booked us in for a visit. But I wanted to meet first to tell you all this. And . . .' We were walking out of the cafe, joining the sea of humanity outside the hospital. 'I wanted to warn you. Layla's a bit different from when you last saw her.'

I nodded.

'Of course she is, she's two years older. But I bet she still likes ponies.'

I had never visited paediatric recuperation before, with its mish-mash of pictures and paintings and toys, designed so that there was something to appeal to every child, whatever their age. The nurse led us past colourful sofas and giant Jenga to a side room. I looked right past a young woman, sitting alone at a table, as my eyes searched for Layla.

'Hi Layla,' said Parminder.

I stared.

The teenager slouched in her chair. She did not look at Parminder or at me, only down at the table. Her hair was long now, hanging limply to her shoulders. A sweater stretched across her wide frame. In fact, she was enormous. And with her size came an almost unnatural stillness. The stillness of a house or a barn or some other huge structure that offers shelter or perhaps a hiding place.

I recalled how the young Layla had sat so childishly on the edge of her seat, slim as a knife, eager to engage, keen for my questions. Her naivety, her animation, her smiles. Could this be the same girl? Round-shouldered. Unable to look at me. Her face almost swallowed by her body and an expression that said she would really like to disappear inside herself.

She was fourteen now. Puberty had evidently arrived late for her, but it was not so much her physical development as her sullen, withdrawn look that shocked me.

'It's good to see you again, Layla,' I said.

She remained silent. She did not look up. She did not move.

I asked: 'How have you been?'

She shrugged.

'Still interested in ponies?'

She shook her head. Not a full shake. Just an intimation.

'You were so passionate about them; specifically, you loved Dartmoor and New Forest ponies best, if I remember rightly.'

She shrugged again. Was she going to speak at all?

It turned out that she wasn't. She studied the floor throughout the time I spent with her. Only her hands moved. As I asked her more questions and tried to engage her in conversation, she knitted, squeezed and twisted her fingers more and more.

I didn't want to retraumatize Layla by asking her to describe again the cruelty that she had experienced. But even very gentle questioning did not elicit a response. I asked her whether she could face the courtroom. She shook her head. It was an answer of sorts. My presence and my questions had distressed her long enough and I got up to go.

'Don't tell me I didn't warn you,' said Parminder as we left the hospital.

I breathed in the fresh air. As is often the way when I'm leaving an institution, it smelled especially good.

'Poor, poor Layla.'

'She's still a sweet girl, really,' Parminder insisted, as if I was arguing with her.

'She didn't meet the threshold for autistic spectrum disorder, but that kid is neurodiverse. And now she's traumatized too.'

Parminder sent me Layla's statement, which described in detail exactly what the girls had done to her. Long afterwards, I could unwillingly recall the small details, like the way one girl had held Layla's arm out while another had lit a match under her fingers. The words they had used. How the branches of some shrub growing in the alley had broken when they pushed her to the ground and one of the girls had picked up the twigs and stuffed them in her mouth and up her nose. How the knife going in had felt like a punch in the stomach. Only the sight of so much blood on her body and on the ground as the older girls left her lying there, only that told her she must have been stabbed.

I wrote a fast report stating clearly that the court should

not retraumatize Layla by asking her to recount her ordeal in public. I was sure they had enough information to prosecute her attacker, perhaps to prosecute all the bullying girls.

Layla did not appear. Parminder rang me from outside the courtroom.

'They were only prosecuting the one who stabbed her: she apparently had a prior conviction for carrying knives. Pleaded guilty. Defence barrister said that an early plea indicated remorse, despite her no comment interview with the police. And he told the court about her difficult childhood. She ended up with just a two-year community order, so she'll soon be back out there.'

'So it's a two-year community order for stabbing and traumatizing Layla?'

'Yep. That's all.'

I looked wordlessly down at my hands. Like one of my own interviewees when perhaps they, too, feel a sense of hopeless despair.

Parminder sighed. We both did. It was hard not to be swamped by feelings of helplessness.

Layla was not abused through physical contact, but Sadie3245 had certainly abused her by sending her the links. Sexual abuse of any kind is a huge, impactful, shocking event in a child's life, and it imprints itself deeply. In the case of pornography, Layla found the material so upsetting that she was drawn back to it again and again for the emotional hit it gave her, no matter how unpleasant that was.

When children have been sexually abused and later start to develop their own sexual fantasies, their minds are likely to return to that emotionally shocking place where they first encountered sex. Pornography is a confusing imprint to return to. And when there has been contact sexual abuse, the most confusing place of all is a victim's feelings about their role in the abuse.

There was certainly a possibility that Layla would become a paedophile, although I thought it unlikely. But that's how others had defined her and how she'd already learned to define herself, and without the right help, that definition might become entrenched. The real criminal, Sadie3245, was, as far as I knew, still out there. He/she had been grooming Layla, that's for sure. Phishing tricks like sending links to children can eventually mean a child will deliver to Sadie3245 the kind of videos the abuser wants to see. These offer a blackmailing opportunity, giving the abuser a still stronger hold over the victim.

But children do not, of course, need a Sadie3245 to view pornography. It is incredible to me that we give our children such easy access to so much. What does it mean for the sex offences of tomorrow if kids watch such extreme material today? I am talking about children looking at porn which features rape and incest and bestiality and extreme violence and more. We take few steps to contain it, but pornography can literally destroy lives. I fear it destroyed Layla's.

37

A formal response to my report on Sally arrived. The phone calls followed.

First came her social worker.

'Has anyone ever suggested,' she said, 'that you lack compassion?'

'No one who knows me. And sometimes the most compassionate thing to do is the hardest.'

'Sally's suffering has been immense and you're suggesting that she should be arrested, charged, perhaps even sent to jail. She doesn't need more suffering!'

'If Sally kills someone, and we both know that she's capable of it, are you suggesting her case shouldn't go through the courts like any homicide?'

'We've never blamed her for anything. We've tried to recognize her particular problems and her parents have certainly given her the love and attention she needs.'

'Sally is causing serious harm to people and her violence is escalating. Love is a wonderful thing, but you can't throw it at kids and hope it will make up for the damage other people have done. She needs to know that there are some boundaries. A multi-agency approach would give her a clear framework. That means, yes, lots of love and healthcare. But it also means police and the justice system. That mixture of kindness and firmness is how we should all try to bring up our children, and in Sally's case, that same mix is needed from the agencies around her.'

'Do you have any children of your own, Dr Harding?'

I paused. 'I am giving you a professional and not a personal opinion.'

'But Sally's own psychiatrist, Dr Weaver – and incidentally she has four children and is very understanding; we think Dr Weaver is a wonderful person – she says that Sally has been so traumatized that she has a desperate need to feel control. We agree with that. We can see her violence is a way of exercising control.'

In her voice was pain, protestation and an edge of anger.

'So you're just going to let her stab people? Even though, as well as hurting others, she retraumatizes herself each time she does it? Please remember, she plans this violence. She is autonomous. Her violence is within the locus of her control. And she's still young enough to learn to control it.'

There was a pause.

'You don't know how hard it's been for our team, for her parents.' She spoke softly. She sounded tired, almost tearful.

She was right. I did not know how hard it was to deal with someone as traumatized as Sally, someone whose past ruled your life, whose violence you dreaded and feared, but whose behaviour you would not proscribe in any way because it came from a place of vulnerability.

'I feel for your whole team and think Sally's parents have been amazing. Wonderful. No criticism is intended. And certainly none is intended of the council either, or her doctors or you social workers. I'm just suggesting you consider thinking a little differently. We know we have a very good Youth Offending Service. They offer amazing practical support: mentorship, training, courses about knife carrying, about violence reduction. They do things with young people that no mental health service can offer. Sally can access that if you're trying to divert her from violence. In my view, both the health and justice systems should work together to give her some more solid boundaries.'

I had not convinced the social worker. I did not convince Sally's psychiatrist, either.

'So you want us to criminalize her? The very thing we've avoided all this time? I thought you'd suggest trauma therapy but instead you've suggested prison!'

'Dr Weaver, you know about the hierarchy of need. Sally can't properly respond to trauma therapy until other more basic needs are met. She is stabbing her carers, which indicates that she doesn't feel safe. So let's meet her first need first: she should feel held and safe within a clear framework.'

'Jail! Is that really the framework you recommend?'

'I hope not. I hope she can be diverted from violence before that question arises. And part of diverting her is for the police to show her where the limits are. At the very least, she needs her own police liaison officer to work with all the other agencies involved. A good, strong liaison officer who wears a helmet, at least metaphorically, can work wonders.'

And of course, Sally's local authority case worker phoned too.

'I am extremely disappointed. Extremely. Sally needs medical help, she should remain in a hospital, she needs a secure mental health unit. And instead you say she should be criminalized? It's outrageous, Dr Harding, and I must inform you that we are considering lodging a formal complaint about you to the GMC.'

'You have no real cause for disappointment. My primary role was to assess her for the presence of mental disorder. I agreed with Dr Weaver that she is not mentally ill. So a forensic health pathway simply would not be right for her. In fact, I think it would just lead to more problems. Children are like sponges, soaking up the maladaptive behaviours and presentations of those around them. It's the wrong environment for Sally. And at the end of the day, there's no acute treatment that will get her out of that place. So what then? She spends the next few years stuck in a forensic mental health system? No, I'm afraid it's not right.'

'I believe she's autistic, whatever you and Dr Weaver say.'

'Even if she were autistic, we couldn't devolve responsibility for her actions on to that, any more than we can blame her early life traumas.'

'Criminalizing the traumatized doesn't help at all. It's positively Victorian. Do you believe in the workhouse too?'

I sighed. No. I did not believe in the workhouse. 'I think everyone needs some boundaries. But when I say that I seem to infuriate people.'

'It infuriates me when you talk about prison!'

'I talk about containment. It's different. Let's pretend for a moment that Sally wasn't adopted by articulate middle-class parents who know how to deal with the system and can demand mental health support. Let's pretend she was left to grow up with her biological parents. I daresay that she would have ended up roaming the streets. I assure you that, here in London, that can happen to very young children. Many of these children become gang members. No one demands an autism assessment for them. No one advocates trauma therapy. Instead, they're seen as just plain bad. They're straight into the criminal justice system. The healthcare system isn't invited to sit by the fire next to criminal justice at any meetings about them. They're marched off to court and then prison.'

There was a long pause.

'I am very pleased . . .' Her voice was stiff. '. . . that, here in our rural county, we were able to find Sally a wonderful placement with loving parents.'

'I'm advocating that, when Sally kicks, she learns that the cot has edges. That's all. I think that your department has done conscientious, caring and outstanding work with Sally and you are to be congratulated. The report says that.'

I had failed to convince the social worker, the doctor or the local authority that there should be a shift in the way Sally was managed. But, of course, I hoped that anyway John Brontë would agree with me.

'Boundaries!' he said, studying his whisky closely, like a patient. 'Why are we so scared of them these days?'

John was more like his old self now. He had written an article about the criminal justice system's misplaced belief in ADHD medication. It had been picked up in the press and he had been widely interviewed. This had boosted his confidence and he had returned to work with new energy and a panic button in his consulting room.

On my arrival today he had grinned broadly. 'I know

how you enjoy your whisky and I've got something wonderful for you to try: it's an outstanding Glenmorangie.'

Yes, I was still pretending to like whisky. Every sip of the Glenmorangie felt as though it was ripping the back of my throat off. But the fire, the whisky, the advice, the wisdom, the laughter: they were all part of the weave of our relationship and I wouldn't take a single thread out.

'One piece of news,' he told me as we sank into our usual seats. 'I was in a secure hospital seeing a teenager and I happened to recognize another patient there. Thomas! Remember him?'

Thomas? The boy who wanted to be a famous serial killer?

'The boy with the screwdriver! We said he was psychotic and got laughed out of court.'

Ouch. I avoided memories of that humiliation.

'He was, indeed, psychotic. He soon had to be transferred to hospital, where apparently they had enormous difficulties stabilizing him. He was finally diagnosed with paranoid schizophrenia.'

'So we were right.'

John smiled. 'I draw small satisfaction from it.'

'I fretted about Thomas a lot,' I confessed.

'Stop all this fretting. I like to think I'm compassionate and that I connect with my patients, but I have a very clear idea of where they end and I begin. Why do you find that so difficult?'

I didn't know the answer but resolved to work harder at staying detached. Then, some time later, another child reappeared from the past and I broke my resolution almost immediately. It was Jessica.

Jessica was the girl who hid in a cupboard while her mother was killed by Jonathan Bowyer. Jessica had so moved me that I had personally intervened to ensure she had professional support. And she had played a huge part in my decision to become a child forensic psychiatrist.

She was dead. She had killed herself.

I was horrified. There was an inquest and I was called to give evidence to the coroner.

A coroner's court is quite different from the Old Bailey. It might be held in modern offices or an ancient function room. Jessica's inquest was held in a town hall, in an ornate ballroom with nineteenth-century oil paintings on the walls. The court felt very temporary: at the weekend, probably this room became a wedding venue. But as a coroner's court enquiring into the suicide of a young girl, it was a joyless place. No one admired the paintings. Jessica's aunt sobbed uncontrollably into a succession of tissues and every witness looked hollow-eyed.

A coroner's job is to ascertain the truth about a death. There is no blame, there are no charges. There is a conclusion – in this case, the conclusion would be suicide – and sometimes a report which can call for scrutiny of a system if the coroner, after hearing all the voices and examining all the evidence, feels the case demonstrates failures.

There were many barristers in court representing many parties – the local Child and Adolescent Mental Health hub as well as the specific staff member who had been seeing Jessica, the aunt, the school . . . there was no jury but still barristers vied to blame each other's clients.

I had to face some aggressive questioning from one, who accused me of interfering. He could not torture me with this possibility more than I had tortured myself. But when the coroner's report finally appeared, I was exonerated: I had simply referred Jessica to local support services and this had no bearing, said the coroner, on her tragic death. I personally held one person responsible for her death: Jonathan Bowyer, the man who had killed her mother. But I did not hear his name mentioned in the courtroom.

38

The child cases I was seeing at that time were varied and interesting, but gang warfare cropped up alarmingly often. A defence lawyer had asked me to write a report on a boy called Eric and he had suggested that Eric might have been overly influenced by the boys who surrounded him. So, on a chilly day in late spring, I waited in a Young Offender Institution to see him. For once, I was not alone. It was visiting time. Here were grandparents in thick coats, a few fathers looking restless and uncomfortable, but, most of all, mothers.

They were sad. No one wants to be visiting their son in an institution because he has committed a crime. Every time a baby is born, we are filled with hope for the future. And where had that hope led these mothers? To sadness, worry and a YOI. There were younger brothers and sisters of offenders here with their parents, and some were babies. The mothers were still reproducing, still hoping.

Hazel and I had been talking a lot about having children. But I could not see past scarred childhoods and damaged lives. And I could not bear the terrible truth that even the most loving and well-meaning parent inevitably and perhaps unknowingly inflicts pain on their child, pain which will stay forever. The responsibilities of parenthood were overwhelming. Hazel knew I felt this way. And, somehow, no baby had arrived.

Prison officers started to lead away the visitors and then I was escorted to the interview area. I could see an angry face, glaring through the small glass window in the first door. The face was shouting something incomprehensible. I hoped that wasn't my client. It was.

Eric was tall and thickset and his face had a very adolescent look of defiance as I sat down opposite him. He was fifteen.

I explained that his solicitor had asked me to come. Eric seemed bored, barely catching my eye, as I went through the formalities. He was looking past me to the noise and people passing outside.

I asked him a series of questions to ascertain that he had the intellectual capacity and mental health to plead. He was able to tell me roughly the role of the judge, what the jury does and what a guilty plea might be.

'Means you done it. You're caught red-handed, innit.'

At that, disconcertingly, he leapt to his feet, eyes wide, hair flying. I recoiled as I awaited his fist but he darted past me to the glass window, pounded on it and yelled something to another lad who was walking by with a prison officer. I could not understand a word. Eric was speaking another language, one which reflected the pecking order here: the lad outside was someone he either dominated or respected, I could not tell which. There's a code and, once they're remanded, young people have to learn it quickly in order to survive.

'You've been in here a few weeks,' I said as he sat down again. 'How have you found it?'

'All right.'

'Do you know anyone from outside?'

'A few. No drama though.'

He sat very still. He may have had the height of a man but, when he assumed no particular expression, I saw the round face of a boy.

'Would you expect drama here?'

'Yeah, there's a few boys from other postcodes. They leave me be.'

'Gangs, you mean?'

He half nodded.

'Are you in a gang, Eric?'

This is a leading question. Very often, kids who insist that they're in gangs are fantasists. Real gang members tend to deny it. But when Eric said that he was a gang member, I did believe him.

Often the vulnerable, the intellectually challenged, or those with mental health problems are easy recruits for gangs to send into other territories to deal drugs. And for the children themselves the lure is great: of belonging, of the glamour of drill music, of the safety and protection of the rest of the gang. Eric did not, however, seem like a vulnerable county-lines kid. And the charges against him far exceeded anything one might expect from such a child.

I asked just a little more, to confirm his fitness to plead.

'What would you do, Eric, if you noticed someone in the jury that you knew? Maybe someone from the past, maybe an enemy.'

Eric narrowed his eyes and shifted them from right to left and back.

'I'd keep my eye on him. Yeah. Nothing gets past me.'

'Do you know what you're charged with?' I asked.

'Yeah. Attempted murder.'

He showed no emotion. He sat back in his chair. I detected something distinct in his manner. I feared it was pride.

'Anything else, Eric?'

'Some drugs stuff too, a bunch of charges.'

'Let's talk about the attempted murder charge. Can you tell me what happened?'

'Well, he was on the bus,' he began. 'I recognized him right away, from another postcode, way across town. He was on his own. Big mistake.'

'So you knew him?'

'I knew him. He stuck me a few weeks ago. In my arm.'

Eric pulled up his left sleeve and showed me a scar on his upper arm. It was obviously a knife wound.

'So I never forget a face,' he said. 'But he didn't remember mine. Not at first, anyway.'

'What happened?'

'He gets on and sits at the front on the top deck. I walk up and block his exit. He acts all big man. Then I get him down on the floor, and he's not so big now, see.' He smiled fleetingly. 'So he's on his back, I'm kneeling over his chest, and I take my blade and I stab him up good.'

'Did he have a blade?'

'I'm not waiting to find out. So I just stab him. Down, down.' He mimed stabbing with alarming realism. 'Down into his face.'

Eric stopped again, distracted by something outside, as though that was much more important than how he had nearly killed someone.

I asked: 'Were you alone, Eric?'

'Yeah. My boys had already got off, we was on the way back from school when he got on the top deck.'

CCTV footage had proved this was untrue but Eric would not betray his mates, whatever the consequences.

'And you're sure this was the boy from the rival gang who'd stabbed you?'

Eric shrugged. His look was one of complete indifference.

'This is important. Are you still sure that the boy you attacked was the boy you thought he was?'

Eric looked around the room. He seemed annoyed.

'I said. I don't forget a face.'

I moved on.

'So what did you do, then, after you'd stabbed him once?'

'Took out his right eye with my second stab, right down to the hilt, easy boy. So now I'm going for his left eye, to blind him proper like, but he puts his hands up, in front of his face like, so the knife stabs through his hands a few times. Then I don't care about his eye anyway, coz now I'm going for his chest.'

No reaction from me. I was listening intently.

'You stabbed his eye and then his chest. What happened?'

'The blade was too short!' He held out his hand, showing me a rough length between two fingers. 'If it was a flick knife he'd be dead for sure, they're this much longer.'

He dropped his hand and stared through the window into the hallway. His face was blank. He showed no emotion at all.

'So why did you stop stabbing him?'

Eric shrugged. 'He goes floppy, I think he's dead, but afterwards I hear he's just pretending. Good move, blud. I get up and run off the bus and ditch the knife.'

Eric's victim had twenty-seven stab wounds. His right optic nerve was severed. He would always be blind in his right eye. He was found not to be carrying a knife. He was not known to be a gang member. He did not live in another postcode. And the CCTV footage showed him looking not aggressive prior to the attack but simply shocked and scared. The police believed that this was a case of mistaken identity. That Eric's victim was not previously known to him. After viewing the footage, I reminded myself yet again always to sit downstairs on buses.

I interviewed Eric for a few hours. I found that his definition of himself was impermeable. He was a tough gang member whom others should respect. He always protected his brothers. And fought his enemies or anyone who was perceived to have slighted him. Little that had happened before he became a gang member had meaning for him. Nothing else really mattered now except his gang brothers and their territory.

Eventually he revealed that he used to enjoy going to a studio for kids where they were encouraged to create their own music but unfortunately it had closed down. And, although he did not know his father, he had heard he was a boxer and had been enthusiastic when a boxing academy was due to open nearby. But it never did.

I remembered how my year off school as a teenager had changed the way I saw myself and the way others saw me. I had spent the time learning the guitar and listening to music, and when I returned to school I was different. I was a musician. I made friends and started bands and the school supported that. I wondered what opportunities had been open to Eric to redefine himself. Maybe if that studio had not closed, or the boxing academy had opened, he would have called himself a singer or a boxer, anyway, not a gang member. And we might not be sitting here now.

I didn't want to believe that this boy was simply bad. I still wanted to believe that everyone was intrinsically good and that there was hope, if not always for adults, for teenagers like Eric at least.

But when I asked Eric if, thinking back, there was anything he would change or do differently, he said this: 'Yeah, oh yeah, I would have waited until he got off the bus and walked up the road behind the boy. What kind of fool would do that in front of the cameras on the bus? The way I should've done it, see, was just a nice and easy stab on the street and walk away, simple boy.'

I told John Brontë about Eric.

'I don't want to believe he's evil,' I said. 'But there were no mental health problems that I could find. No trauma or abuse or real deprivation. Gang thinking has taken him over. But unless we blame the gang, there's no explanation for his complete lack of remorse except . . .'

John was quick.

'He's showing some psychopathic traits, but for God's sake don't call him a psychopath at fifteen!'

'It's not just Eric. Where is this gang thinking coming from? There are kids stabbing other kids out there every day.'

'For them, there's a war on,' said John. 'Society's norms all fall by the wayside and the gangs develop their own codes of conduct: it's the rule of war. They carry out terrible atrocities under some mass ideological construct. What our young people need is a sense of belonging in society, ownership of the world in which they live. They need access to a lot more activities, sport, drama, anything that will involve them. I remember there used to be music studios for young people in London's most deprived areas and thousands of children passed through them, finding their voice and a passion in life, directing their energies into something positive, prosocial and fulfilling. More exciting than a gang. More exciting than crime. They were provided with the gift of music, one that will stay with them forever.'

'Did all the studios close?' I asked miserably.

'Every one of them, for lack of funds. No one wanted to invest in our children.'

I sighed.

'So what can I do about Eric?'

'Nothing. I know you like to play the saviour but this is society's wider problem. You'll just have to tell his solicitor that you couldn't find any psychiatric defence for him and then move on.'

We paused and gulped at our whisky. Scrape, burn in my throat.

'What can we do for these young people?'

'Us? Nothing. Society as whole? Develop some proper structures for them instead of chucking them out of mainstream school and mainstream society.'

'Eric had a record as long as your arm; he probably should have been locked up a long time ago,' I said sadly. 'People start yelling about criminalizing children, but if something had been done earlier, he could have been offered new, different ways to define himself.'

John nodded agreement. 'Must be exhausting playing the tough guy. I daresay there are times when Eric would love to be someone else.'

We were silent then, because we knew it was probably too late for Eric. He had committed a crime of the utmost violence and he would spend years in the kind of jail which simply nurtured the battlelines of the streets.

Whenever I interviewed kids like Eric, it made me sure of one thing. I certainly did not want to bring a baby into such a violent world. Obviously, it was impossible to keep a child safe. I resolved to tell Hazel that very evening that I categorically believed it would be wrong to have a baby and there was no point discussing it any more.

When I returned home, she said: 'You've been with John.'

'How did you know?'

'You smell of whisky.'

She looked lovely. Radiant. Usually the smell of whisky would make her turn away but now she did not move.

She said: 'I've got some news.'

I looked at her smile: broad. Her eyes: shining. Her face: soft. And guessed at once what that news was.

I had resolved that our violent world was no place for a child and I had been certain for many years that I was not father material. Why, then, did I find myself beaming back at my wife with a smile so immense, so wide, so completely beyond my control and so unceasing that my face started to ache?

39

The police rang me to ask if I would write a psychiatric report on a young murder suspect. His name was Liam. His defence team had instructed a psychiatrist, who had produced a robust report arguing that Liam had been psychotic at the time of the homicide. He would plead not guilty to murder and guilty only to manslaughter with diminished responsibility.

Liam had driven his aunt to a remote spot and then strangled her before pushing her into a pond. She had not drowned: the pathologist said that she was already dead before she hit the water.

I interviewed Liam in his secure unit and detected no mental illness at all and certainly no psychosis. His 999 call and police bodycam footage from immediately after the crime confirmed this for me. Miss Swinney's death appeared to be calculated and planned. I feared that Liam was a very dangerous young man.

So, the case – murder or manslaughter? – hinged on the testimony of two psychiatrists.

While Hazel grappled with the tiredness of early pregnancy, reports pinged backwards and forwards between me and the defence psychiatrist, Dr Graf. He was sceptical of every word I wrote and his team insisted on seeing my notes. Notes I had made during the interview with Liam and after it, notes from meetings with his parents. Nothing was enough for them. What had I scribbled as I read his school reports? They demanded notes of notes of notes. Our correspondence dragged on for months. Hazel's belly swelled.

'It's the most aggressive defence ever,' I told her as we waited for a scan. 'They're trying to catch me out and expose me as a charlatan in court.'

Hazel laid her hands on the baby. I could see him kicking inside her. 'Something about you seems to make other people aggressive,' she said.

'Harding, please!' called the sonographer.

A few minutes later, Liam was forgotten. So were all my cases. There, on the screen, kicking without a care in the world, was a tiny boy. Our son. Hazel and I looked at the screen and looked at each other and back at the screen. I felt a mixture of joy and dread. Very soon, we would see him in three dimensions. We would hold him close. So much that was wonderful lay ahead. So much that could go wrong.

Liam's case reached court soon afterwards. The room was packed with his relatives. The press sat in rows.

The defence psychiatrist, Dr Graf, gave evidence over several days. Then it was my turn. We broke for the weekend. And now here we were again. The same court, the same barristers, the same judge, the same psychiatrists, the same defendant, the same jury. Only the weather outside was different: the temperature had dropped below freezing now and the streets were icy.

The judge had told me on Friday that the court would expect an explanation from me. If Liam wasn't psychotic, why did he kill his aunt?

I had spent the weekend agonizing over how to frame my answer. I knew I could not produce something as simple, clear-cut and easily defined as that single word: psychosis. The truth was so much more complex. It could not be packaged. It would not be welcomed. It might not be understood: not by me, not by anyone, perhaps not even by Liam.

I waited outside the courtroom as everyone filed in ahead of me until I was left alone in the silent corridor. I rocked my ankles while I waited to be called. Finally, the court clerk appeared and asked me to enter. I took my place at the witness stand, feeling all eyes upon me like an actual, physical weight as I arranged my papers in front of me.

The defence barrister stood, put his hands behind his back, and looked thoughtful.

'Dr Harding, you dismiss the possibility of psychosis. You state that Liam was not mentally ill when he killed his aunt. However, you have as yet given no alternative explanation for his behaviour. I invite you to do so now.'

I paused.

'I don't know why Liam killed his aunt. The only person to know that is Liam himself.'

His withering glance at the jury invited them to agree that this was completely inadequate.

'You don't know. And yet you continue to insist that he was not psychotic?'

'I found no evidence for psychosis at the time of the incident.'

'You cannot find any alternative explanation, yet you remain certain that Dr Graf's perfectly understandable explanation is wrong?'

'No one knows what happened for certain. I am giving my opinion, based on the evidence I've seen, and my assessment of Liam.'

'I see.' He paused and looked significantly, almost conspiratorially, at the jury before turning back to me. 'You did mention a temper tantrum last week, Dr Harding. Anger, then. Do you propose that as a reason Liam killed his aunt?'

'In my view he was angry,' I said. 'There is evidence of anger. But I don't know that is the reason.'

The barrister's eyes ran along the row of jury members, as though he were sweeping their faces into a net. Then, when he had caught them all, he turned back to me.

'Do you really think it is realistic to suggest that a temper tantrum might account for a killing of this nature, Dr Harding?'

'Anger is a powerful emotion,' I said. 'I don't know if anger accounts for it, but it may well be a factor.'

'Indeed. But a tantrum! Over a mobile phone, no less.' He gave the jury a glance to show how absurd this was. 'So, apart from that, you propose no other motive?'

'Anger could certainly contribute to risk,' I said, 'and I think that there was a melting pot of risk that led to the incident . . .'

He jumped in quickly.

'We're not interested in hearing any speculative theories. We want facts here, and obviously we expect those facts to be very firmly based on evidence. Do you understand your duty, Dr Harding?'

This was a blatant attack on my credibility. I felt myself redden.

'Yes,' I said, trying to make my voice firm.

'When Dr Graf gave evidence in this court, he did deal with the possibility that anger might have been a motive. He described it as absurd. Inconceivable that a child would kill someone he loved because he was angry about a mobile phone. Did you hear that evidence, Dr Harding?'

Yes, I had heard the defence dismiss the possibility that Liam had acted in anger. Of course. Anger, callous indifference, frustration, selfishness, loneliness . . . admitting the involvement of human emotions in all their complexity would have conceded that Liam might be responsible for his actions and could have committed murder.

'Indeed, as you will recall, Dr Graf stated here that the nature of the crime itself, the violence against a loved one, the unusual circumstances, the call to the police; all this was further evidence that Liam was psychotic at the time of the killing. As Dr Graf said, how can Liam *not* have been mentally ill to do these things?'

I dragged myself away from the barrister and faced the jury. Two rows of faces turned to me.

'I can understand that it is difficult for us to accept that a child who is not mentally ill might kill a loved relative. I understand how difficult it is for us to accept that a child can do such a thing when sane, by choice. But that is the unfortunate conclusion I have come to. I searched carefully for evidence of psychosis at the time of the killing and found none. Liam has not become psychotic since this assault. Indeed, he has never been treated for psychosis, when one might expect psychosis at the time of the death to have developed afterwards into further psychotic illness. It did not. Liam is not mentally ill now. In my view, mental illness is not a reasonable explanation for Miss Swinney's killing.'

'Excuse me, Dr Harding,' said the judge. 'It would be helpful for myself and the jury if you could please try to answer the question. If not mental illness, why did Liam kill his aunt? Are you saying he killed in anger? Or not?'

'We can't reduce such a serious incident to a choice between anger and psychosis. I understand the need to know and I am trying to assist the court and jury as best I can. But I don't know what drove Liam to kill his aunt. I do think he was angry with her and that may have been one factor. But, most importantly, I don't find evidence of him suffering from psychotic illness. Indeed, in my view there were signs of planning. The presence and use of a dog lead, for example, when there was no dog. The call to the emergency services was clear and rational. He was interviewed later that day by a mental health practitioner and found to be not psychotic. He was interviewed the next day in court and found to be not psychotic. He has not developed a subsequent psychotic illness and has never been treated with anti-psychotic medication. I do not find evidence for a mental disorder that substantially diminished his responsibility for his actions that day. From this, it is only possible to draw one conclusion. In my opinion, Liam made a choice. He decided to kill his aunt, he planned to kill his aunt, and he did kill her. That was his choice and he is responsible for making it. Not a mental illness. Liam.'

The judge held my gaze and then looked down to make notes. Did he seem disappointed? Perhaps.

'Children can make bad decisions,' I added. 'Children can do bad things. It's hard for us to recognize that. We might not want to believe that Liam did the worst possible thing of all. We might prefer to be comforted by the belief that his bad decisions were driven by trauma or mental illness or anything except the boy himself. But . . . I'm sorry I can't offer that comfort. Because there is no evidence for it.'

'Thank you, Dr Harding,' said the defence barrister, frowning, dissatisfied, shaking his head just a little. 'I have no further questions for you.'

I left the court. I had offered the jury all I could: now it was for them to decide which psychiatrist they believed.

Choice and autonomy are our currency in life. We make choices that dictate our journey ahead and we must take responsibility for those choices. We might become ill, perhaps mentally ill, and our ability to make good decisions might be impaired. But as a society we can't assume that extreme behaviours result solely from illness or trauma, however incomprehensible they may appear.

Equally, we can't assume some people are simply 'evil'. The human condition is more complicated than that, and life rarely, if ever, fits into a dichotomy of good versus evil, mad versus bad, however our legal system might be set up.

Rather than reducing extreme behaviours into a palatable dichotomy, we must listen carefully to the voices of those who harm us and decide the degree of autonomy and responsibility they must take for their actions. We must remain open, curious, and hold the pendulum in the middle. In my experience, there is never an easy answer. Only shades of grey.

Liam would take his place in my memory soon and I

would be immersed again in other cases. These days, they came at me in an endless stream. So many young faces before me: dour, sad, angry, hurt, confused. And all of them, even the most violent and scary, so vulnerable. Most of them let down, now or earlier, by the adults around them. Some without adults at all. What a vast sea of children there seemed to be out there. And here I was bringing another child into the dangerous ocean.

The day after I had finished giving evidence at Liam's trial, Hazel and I made our way through the icy streets to the hospital. Knowing that, when we left it, there would be another human in this world and it would be for us to love, protect, guide and parent him.

I was still haunted by fears: could I really keep my son safe here in London when so many children were simply not safe at all? Could I really be trusted not to turn into my father, identifying with the violent abuser after all these years? And what about the tricky question of introducing and maintaining boundaries? It was easy to criticize others, but would I be able to show my own child the edges of the cot firmly and with kindness?

As we waited – for a midwife, for a bed, for a baby – my phone rang. I was sure Hazel did not want me to answer but I saw the call came from the detective who had been in charge of Liam's case. This must mean there was a verdict.

Hazel looked distressed. 'Duncan, couldn't you just stop working for one morning?'

Too late.

'Hello?'

The detective's voice was familiar. 'Okay, we have a verdict and I'm afraid the jury agreed with Dr Graf. They found Liam not guilty of murder.'

I felt no surprise, just something sinking in my chest.

'They went for manslaughter with diminished responsibility. Sorry, Duncan. I know you worked hard on this case.'

Manslaughter. I had let the world down. If only I'd been better, explained things more clearly. But I had to remind myself that, ultimately, the court is always right. I spoke for just a couple of days but the jury had sat through weeks of forensic evidence: coroner's reports, crime scene photographs, body-worn camera footage. They had a much fuller view of the case and I had to trust that they had made the right decision. Except that . . . perhaps, like so many others, they had not been ready to believe that a child could be guilty of murder. Maybe they had chosen that verdict because they simply preferred to believe Liam's violence was driven by mental illness rather than by his own choices. That he was sick rather than dangerous.

Watched by a sad Hazel, I received the thanks of the police officer.

'Any chance that you could turn your phone off now?' she asked when the call was over and a midwife was beckoning to us. We stood up. The courtroom, the barristers, Liam, all disappeared from my head as suddenly as if they had fallen into a mineshaft. We were going to have a baby!

And now I was swamped with fears. Not the low-level anxieties that had nagged me for years about fatherhood, but huge fears, towering like enormous waves. Would

Hazel be all right? Would the baby be all right? Would everything be all right?

It was.

Later that day, by Hazel's side, I held our baby in my arms for the first time.

I experienced a rush of joy and love so powerful and so pure that it inhabited my entire body, soul and mind. Nothing I had imagined could have prepared me for this. There was nothing else to think, to feel. There was only this baby. No reasoning, no worrying, no background noise. Just a tiny, wonderful, heart-stopping scrap of humanity.

A few hours later, I livestreamed pictures from the hospital to my mother. Once she was satisfied that George the cat was safely installed with the neighbours, she had agreed to live in a care home. Because her cancer had cheated us all. It had advanced stealthily, suddenly, lethally.

'Here he is!' I cried. Hazel's tired, happy face. The baby kicking, staring around at his new world.

A carer held up the screen for her and I watched my mother carefully.

She looked hard for a moment. She frowned with concentration. And then a wonderful thing happened. A smile, the first for many months. Broad, simple, unalloyed. Our baby had effortlessly brought her something I had so often tried to deliver. For a moment, as her life was drawing to a close, her grandson had made my mother happy.

I turned back to the baby to wonder at his fingers, his toes, to gaze at his face, to feel astonished by him. Most of all I was filled with a new and profound sense of focus. So now I understood. Now my professional life informed the personal at the deepest level. Now I could see at last what life is about.

It's about loving a child, loving children.

It's about providing a safe space where they can trust the world around them, explore, develop their own thoughts and find their place.

It's about young people discovering their true voice and knowing that someone is listening to them.

It's about hearing that voice, even when it hurts to listen.

It's about ensuring young people can find safe spaces outside the home, especially if home offers no safety: places they can go to make music, play games, build dreams.

It's about boundaries, the boundaries all of us, family and society, can show each child kindly.

It's about accepting the unpalatable truth that children can do bad things and that even this must be heard. And that the child's behaviour must be recognized and contained by all of us to help that young person find their path.

It's about understanding that we want to care for, treat and hug our children, but sometimes they need more than family, health, social care and education. When needs are complex, then complex solutions may be required. And that solution might include the police, the justice system, and, yes, perhaps even custody. It's about knowing this is not criminalization. It is kindness. It is support. It is love.

It's about my child. It's about your child. And children unknown. It's about all our children.

Acknowledgements

A career is built upon foundations laid by others, and I'm profoundly grateful to all the clinicians, mentors, colleagues, patients and families I have learned from for all these years.

Many thanks to my agent, Luigi Bonomi, without whom this book would not exist. Thanks also to Rowland White, Ariel Pakier and the team at Michael Joseph, who have stood by me and helped mould my life and career into these pages.

None of this would be possible without the love and support of my wife and son.

My mum died before this book was published, so she never saw this in print. I am so grateful for everything she gave me in life, and the opportunities she unlocked. I wish I could call her again and tell her that.

I have a sister but chose not to mention her in this book, to protect her privacy.